Clean Eating Alice

Eat Well
Every Day

Thorsons
An imprint of HarperCollins*Publishers*
1 London Bridge Street
London SE1 9GF

www.harpercollins.co.uk

First published by Thorsons 2016

10 9 8 7 6 5 4 3 2

Photography © Martin Poole
Food styling: Kim Morphew
Prop styling: Wei Tang
Hair and make-up: Sharon Massey

A catalogue record of this book is available from
the British Library

ISBN 978-0-00-816723-3

Printed and bound by GPS Group

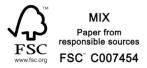

MIX
Paper from
responsible sources
FSC™ C007454
www.fsc.org

FSC™ is a non-profit international organisation established to promote the
responsible management of the world's forests. Products carrying the FSC
label are independently certified to assure consumers that they come from
forests that are managed to meet the social, economic and ecological needs
of present and future generations, and other controlled sources.

Find out more about HarperCollins and the environment at
www.harpercollins.co.uk/green

All recipes are based on fan-assisted oven temperatures. If you
are using a conventional oven, raise the temperature 20°C higher
than stated in recipes.

The nutrition and health claims made in this book have all been
checked by a registered food nutritionist. All recipes labelled
as healthy have been checked to ensure that they are not overly
indulgent and that they do contain ingredients with levels of
micronutrients that warrant an EU registered nutrition claim.
All nutrition claims relating to ingredients themselves have
been checked and any health claims made have been researched
and do not state fact but indicate that this is what the research
suggests. Recipes have been labelled if they are gluten free (GF),
dairy free (DF) or vegetarian (V). These checks have been done
based on the average ingredients of products on the market and
assuming those who are gluten free will use gluten-free versions
of ingredients such as oats, stock etc. For anyone who is coeliac,
it is the responsibility of the individual to double check labels of
ingredients before making recipes. Refer to page 43 for advice on
ensuring a balanced and healthy fat intake.

It is recommended that readers always consult a qualified medical
specialist for individual advice. This book should not be used as
an alternative to seeking specialist medical advice, which should
be sought before any action is taken. The author and publishers
cannot be held responsible for any errors and omissions that may
be found in the text, or any actions that may be taken by a reader
as a result of any reliance on the information contained in the
text, which is taken entirely at the reader's own risk.

Clean Eating Alice

Eat Well Every Day

Nutritious, healthy recipes for life on the go

Thorsons

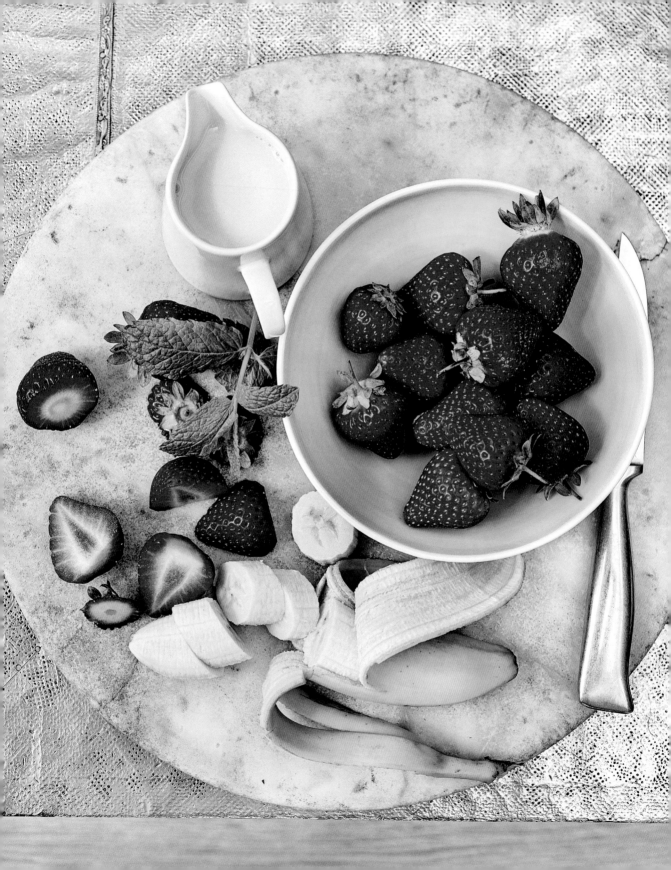

CONTENTS

INTRODUCTION 6

NUTRITION 36

BREAKFAST 52

LUNCH 88

DINNER 118

SNACKS 154

PLATES 180

MEAL PLANNER 206

CONVERSION CHARTS 216

INDEX 218

ACKNOWLEDGEMENTS 223

INTRODUCTION

For those of you familiar with my story, you'll know that I spent the majority of my teenage years buying in to dangerous quick-fix diets.

This entailed restrictive eating, cutting out food groups and believing that slogging away on a treadmill was the only way to keep fit and lose weight. The world we now live in constantly encourages us to believe that we need to make drastic changes and restrict ourselves in pursuit of a healthy physique.

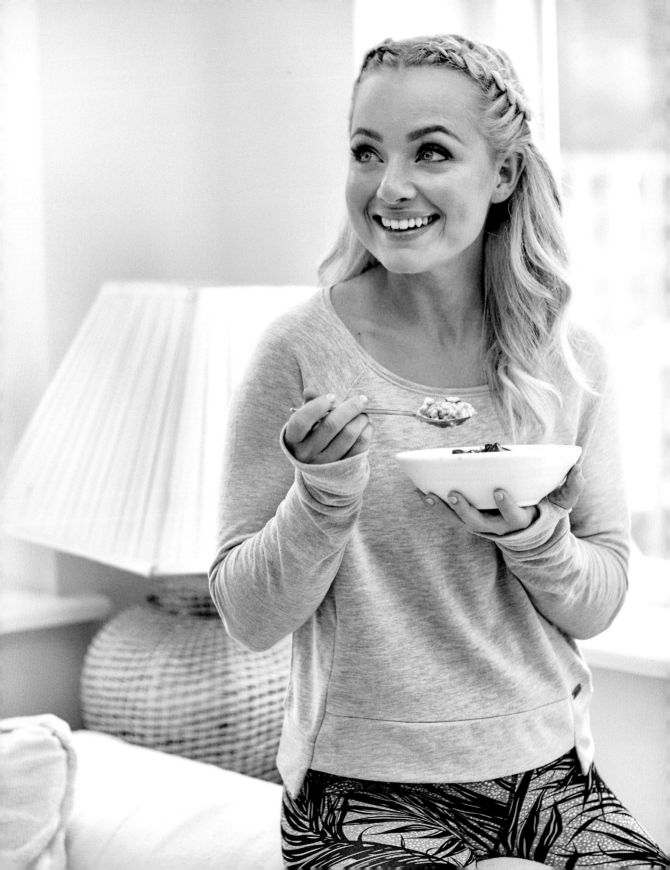

'STOP BEING AFRAID OF WHAT COULD GO WRONG AND FOCUS ON WHAT COULD GO RIGHT.'

The food industry is full of conflicting statements that can leave you totally perplexed as to what is actually good for you and what isn't. If you believed every report written, it's likely you'd end up allowing yourself a controlled list of foods you could count on one hand. Having been there, and been baffled by the amount of confusing information there was, I know how hard it is. Every 'diet' has a different angle, whether it is 'cutting out carbs', 'low-fat' or 'juicing', and I was left searching but failing to find anything that simply promoted a sustainable, balanced and inexpensive approach to achieving a year-round healthy lifestyle. The key for me was to find a way of life that allowed me to eat delicious, easy-to-make food all of the time. The emphasis had to be on fresh and accessible ingredients and dishes that worked for everyday life, be it quick lunches on the go, post-workout breakfasts or simple but delicious dinners. What I wanted to showcase were all the physical and mental benefits of being healthy.

In my first book, I shared how I began on my own journey, developing a way of eating and a lifestyle that meant I no longer found myself going round and round on the diet 'roundabout', which messed about not only with my body but also with my mind. Those of you who have followed me through Instagram will know that that is simply not the case any more. I have transformed both mentally and physically, becoming the strong, healthy and confident woman that I'd always dreamed of being. And now, I am championing what I feel is a much-needed breath of fresh air into what I think is an incredibly saturated market. One of the most valuable things I learnt on my journey was that, to create the most lasting and impactful change, you must first start with the right environment in which to make that change. You have to know that you want to commit to eating to fuel both body and mind, and this book is designed to help you take the first steps and then go on to make it a permanent way of life.

After talking you through my approach, I will examine the basics of nutrition to help you understand what bodies need and why, so that you can make educated choices for yourself rather than having to religiously follow a 'plan'.

After that comes the food section of recipes. Then I will help guide you on how to build the perfect plate, with the right balance of foods to fuel you both mentally and physically.

TAKING THE FIRST STEPS

We could tell ourselves that we are going to begin our journey every single day, and yet that very rarely happens. Life gets in the way, birthdays happen, holidays happen, and suddenly we are a month, two months, a year later and have made no change. Now I'm not going to sit here and wag my finger at you; believe me when I say I am the first to discourage that prescriptive style of helping you achieve your goal. But what I will say is that there really is no better time to start than now. We're creatures of habit, and change is going to feel weird. The first week, month or few months may feel difficult, and require a little hard work, but I believe that is only because you are undoing years of daily habits that have brought you to where you are today. While I'm not going to fob you off by saying that creating a total lifestyle change is going to be a walk in the park, what I will do is help you implement some everyday tools and techniques that will allow you to create a seamless transition into healthier, happier living.

These tools aren't miraculous exercises or superfoods that will somehow transform your physique, but rather are small lifestyle changes that I feel are essential in establishing the most stable platform from which you can then progress your journey. It is all about making your own decisions and understanding what food is good for you and how to make sure you eat right every day.

For the first week, I am not going to encourage any changes within your diet or exercise regime, I just want you to focus in on yourself and encourage you to become aware of your daily habits. Becoming more aware of, and tuning into, your body seems silly, but can often be key in understanding why you may be held back from achieving your desired goal. For example, many studies have shown the benefits of getting a good amount and quality of sleep and the correlation this has to weight loss, and yet this key aspect of our lifestyle is so often overlooked by many 'diets'. I want to encourage you to not focus solely on diet or exercise, as I feel that they are only small pieces of a bigger picture. Try thinking about a few of the questions below, and perhaps keep a diary for this week to help you better understand your body and mind, and how they may be affecting your choices:

• What and when are you eating?
• How does this make you feel?
• Are you drinking enough water?
• Are you getting decent sleep?
• How much are you moving throughout the day?
• Are you feeling stressed?
• Have you exercised today?
• If so, how did that make you feel?

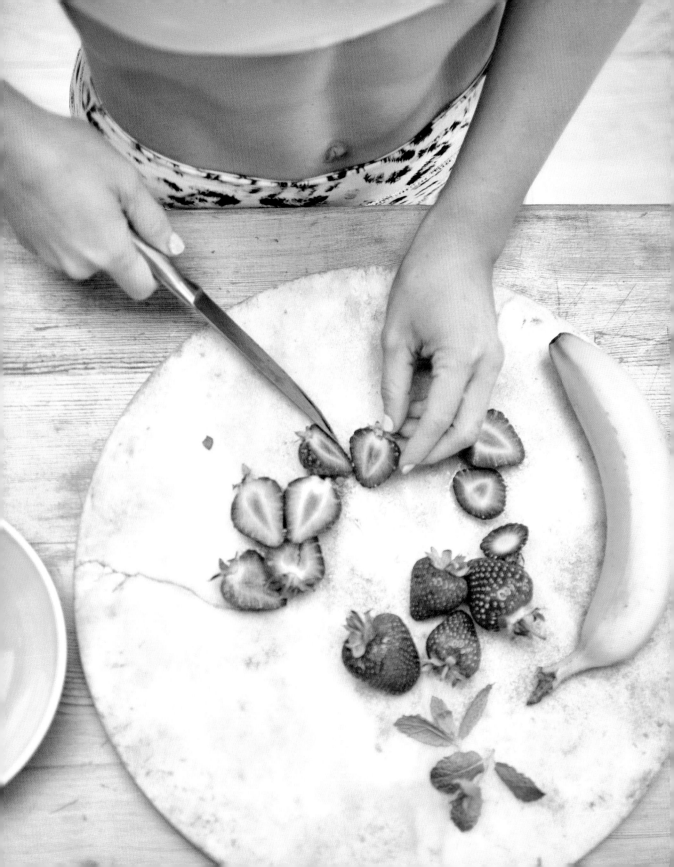

I see our bodies as a pyramid. I know first hand that we cannot solely focus on changing one aspect of our bodies without stepping back and working on the bigger picture in order to establish the most lasting change.

Move

I am not a hardline personal trainer who is going to insist that you work out for hours on end or go to the gym every day. That isn't always healthy, nor is it sustainable – and most of all, it isn't a realistic approach to exercise. And I am a realist; I know how busy life can be and that fitting in exercise is something that can often fall to the bottom of the list when other things take over. My advice here would be not to panic about having to take exercise, but just get started by gradually increasing your daily activity levels – perhaps by walking to work a few days a week, going for a brisk walk in your lunch break or generally being more active throughout your day. All of this will mean you increase your energy expenditure without even stepping into a gym.

To make exercise a part of your routine, you need to find an activity that *you* enjoy. I began weight training and I found instantly that it was something I felt engaged in and so I was motivated to get stronger, but I know this doesn't happen for everyone. Whether it's Zumba, aerobics, swimming or cycling, if you want to achieve long-term change it is important to find a way of getting moving that you love, then incorporate that into your week in a realistic timetable. I hope with my first book, *The Body Bible*, you will also see how simple it can be to do a good workout in the comfort of your own home.

If you are really struggling with motivation, try purchasing a step counter so that you can see how active you are throughout the day; seeing the numbers in front of you might inspire you to keep moving and increase your exercise level. Partnering up with a workout buddy is also an excellent way of motivating both parties to work out. And finally, setting goals – both short- and long-term – can help you to keep on track with your exercise regime.

Mind

It is my honest belief that no lasting changes can take place until you are in a positive place in which you can then establish your new lifestyle. It sounds a little clichéd, but I feel that, before physical changes can be seen, the biggest change needs to occur in the mind. You want to establish a good relationship with your body whereby you feel as though you are making changes not because you hate the shape you are in, but because you want to become the healthiest, happiest version of yourself possible. We are constantly encouraged to compare ourselves to others and to idolise celebrity bodies in glossy magazines and on social media, and this allows us to become disheartened with the package we are given, driving us to believe that we need to make drastic changes in order to achieve our desired physique. I hope that reading this book and following my Instagram encourages you to divert your mind to focusing on the fact that healthy looks different on every body, there is no one desired physique and your goal should ultimately be health *and* happiness: neither one should be sacrificed to achieve the other. I want this book to inspire a love of food and creating recipes that you enjoy cooking. A big motivator for me when I started on this path was to savour the excitement I felt watching the food I cooked take shape into a delicious-looking plate I knew was doing me good.

Food

This was the biggest change for me, and the third element of our pyramid. Food is such an integral part of us, and the thing we often find the most difficult to change for a lasting period of time. We develop habits from a young age that then carry us through our lives and are often quite difficult to undo, and I know first hand that by creating healthy habits that you incorporate into your day-to-day routine, eating well will slowly become second nature to you, resulting in a lasting and sustainable change. What must be understood here is that nutrition isn't 'one size fits all'. It's incredibly complex and requires you to make decisions based on your own body and not because it worked for X or Y, so therefore it must work for you. That is why I haven't created a 'plan' or 'six weeks to fab' book where I promise you rock-hard abs in a given period of time. That is *not* me. What I can deliver on is a book full of nutritionally dense recipes that you can incorporate into *your* own healthy balanced life. Your choices. Your goals. Your body. I'm just here to kick-start your motivation and inspiration, and be your pocket personal trainer and cheerleader along the way.

FOREVER

So now you've spent your first week identifying small changes you can make to your lifestyle, you are hopefully feeling slightly more in control.

'The happiest people don't have the best of everything, they just make the best of everything.'

You've identified some good foundations from which you can begin to incorporate sustainable changes to your lifestyle. But first, let me explain where my approach comes from. The world we live in constantly instils in us that instant gratification is the norm. We have become accustomed to everything happening at the click of our fingers and you only need to flick through a few glossy magazines to be told that you can get abs in six weeks, and that diet shakes will apparently provide you with the correct nourishment over real food. I've spoken at length throughout my journey about how drastic diets and extreme measures – the whole 'no pain no gain' approach, although they may be incredibly motivating in the short term and provide quick results, simply aren't sustainable for a long period of time. In my opinion, they can be mentally and physically damaging.

Dieting on very low calories is likely to leave you with some sort of nutritional deficiency. It's incredibly difficult to consume enough of all the vital macro and micronutrients you need for basic health and hormonal function when you are restricting yourself in this extreme way. Your body can take a real hit, and dramatically reducing your calories creates an increase in the body's production of the hormone ghrelin, as well as others. These hormones are the hunger hormones, sending signals to your brain to tell you you're hungry. This therefore can mean that as soon as the 'diet' ends, you can feel an excessive desire to eat more than you need, therefore succumbing to a rebound period in which binging or over-eating can then occur, creating the yo-yo diet effect that we so often see.

Most importantly, the most worrying result of these crash diets is the effect they have on your relationship with food. It is my belief that food isn't just fuel; it should be enjoyed and not just seen as sustenance. Entertaining fad diets or low-calorie restriction merely serves the purpose of showing that if you eat a very small amount of food you will achieve fat loss – but what lessons are then learned? Seeing quick results can often lead you to then fear increasing your calories once a plan has finished, resulting in a cycle of miserable restriction. It isn't normal and it can't last; we need good food to survive and thrive. One thing I want each and every one of you to tell yourself on a daily basis while using this book is that: *You are in this for the long term.* If you truly want to make change, forget magic-wand quick fixes and place your energies in believing that slow and steady changes, where you learn to eat in a sustainable, flexible and *enjoyable* manner, will ultimately provide you with the healthiest and longest-lasting results. It will allow you to eat a varied diet – full of goodness, but full of interesting food combinations so that you never feel bored or uninspired to try something new.

Over the next few pages I will share my top tips for week two and beyond. This is where we want to begin to make small changes to enable lifelong results. Write these down in your diary, stick them on your fridge or pop them next to your bed, so that you are gently reminding yourself of this week's goals.

1

Create a morning routine

It is my belief that the morning is a pivotal time of the day; if we can have a good start, we are far more likely to make good choices throughout the rest of the day, too.

Although at first it may seem as if a little extra effort is required, establishing a consistent morning routine means that it will soon become second nature for you to implement your healthy habits, such as preparing your overnight oats and enjoying them when you wake up, instead of starting every day with that morning panic that means you begin your day stressed.

For the first few weeks of making a lifestyle change, it's incredibly useful to set an alarm and get up at the same time every morning – this will allow plenty of time to prepare breakfast. To implement more structure into your mornings, try writing yourself a timeline for the first few weeks, and pop it on the fridge or by your bed. Mine would look a little like the list below, but it's important to make it personal to you, ensuring that you allow enough time to complete each task without running around like a headless chicken.

1. Wake up, drink a glass of water.
2. Read a few pages of a book (10 mins).
3. Get up, prepare breakfast (15 mins).
4. Shower, dress, make-up (30 mins).
5. Leave the house.

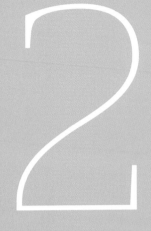

2

Set short- and
long-term goals,
both physically
and mentally

When I speak to people who want to instigate a change in their physique, I always find that their focus rests solely on their exterior. Very few acknowledge that the biggest change to occur is often in the mind, which will in turn help to create physical change.

As I'm sure many of you can relate to, developing a healthy relationship with food and with your body isn't the easiest of tasks, but I feel that incorporating both mind and body goals into your lifestyle change ensures that you're constantly striving to achieve the balanced pyramid approach, as discussed previously, and you aren't neglecting one aspect of what is a much bigger picture.

There are so many ways to set goals, but I often find that writing them down in a journal is a really nice and personal way of remembering them.

I also find that being organised with your food often increases motivation, and establishes a consistent routine that you are able to follow with very little effort. Planning your meals for the week ahead on a Sunday, for example, will help you to avoid those days where you search the cupboards for random ingredients to throw together when you get in late from work. It is then that you can often find yourself making the wrong choices.

Creating a shopping list and a food planner for the week is the perfect way to get into a habit of organising your meals for the week ahead, budgeting to ensure you don't spend a fortune on food each week, and keeping your motivation high, as you have delicious planned meals to look forward to cooking and eating.

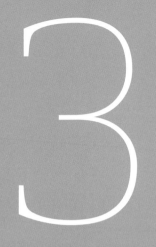

3

Make simple swaps

As talked about a lot in *The Body Bible*, it's my mission to show you that healthy eating doesn't have to mean drastic change; making simple swaps within your diet can often make a huge difference.

With the varied number of recipes supplied in both this book and *The Body Bible*, I hope I can show you how realistic it can be to totally overhaul your diet by making simple swaps so that you don't feel as though you're sacrificing your favourite foods. For this second week, the simple swaps are of even more importance as you begin to make change. While you are adopting a new way of eating, it's important that you try to create as seamless a transition as possible and, by simply swapping like for like, you can still feel as though you're enjoying the foods you once did; it's just that now they're packed full of a lot more goodness.

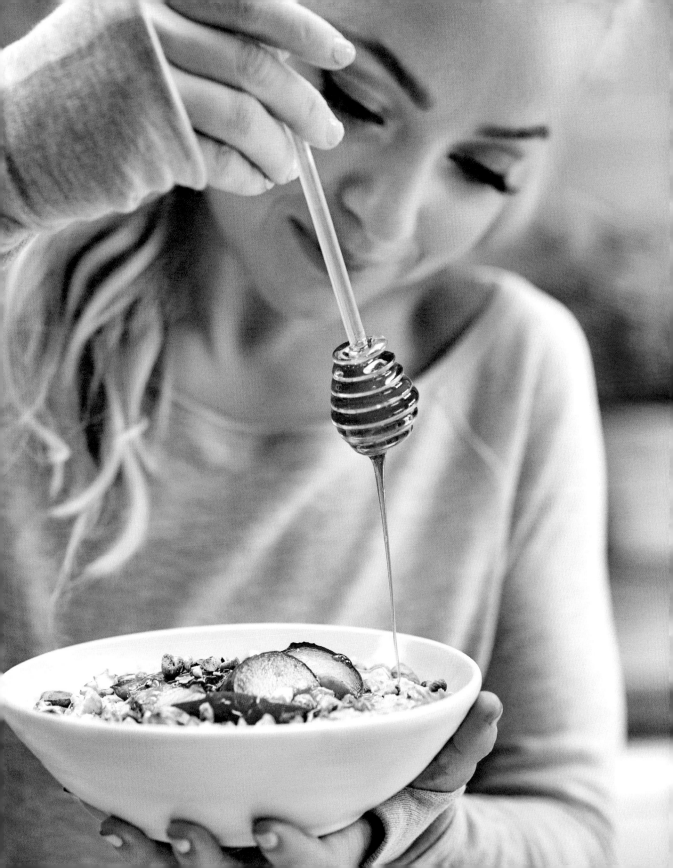

Examples of some simple swaps:

Cereal
vs
Oats

Breakfast
bars
vs
Energy
balls

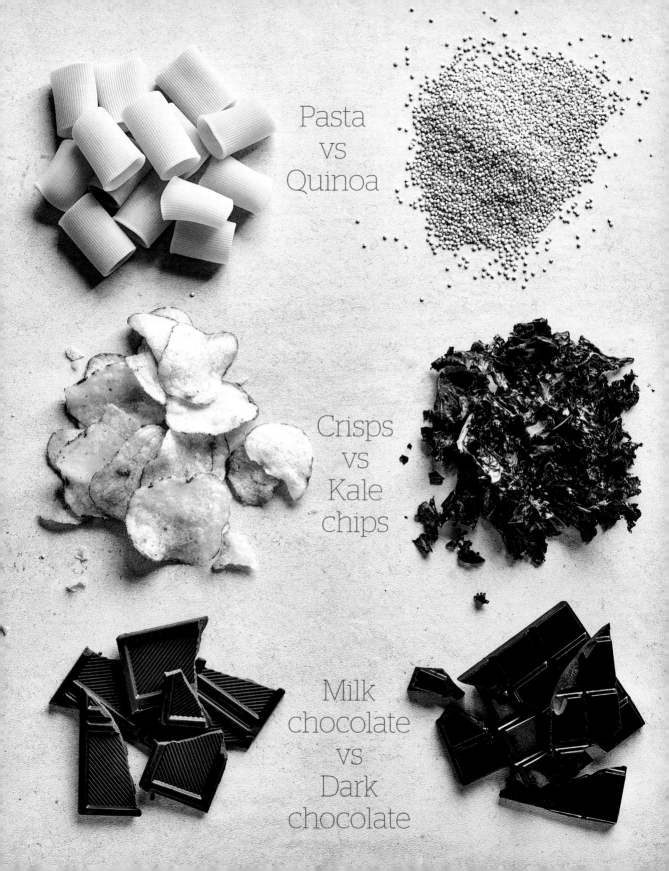

Pasta
vs
Quinoa

Crisps
vs
Kale
chips

Milk
chocolate
vs
Dark
chocolate

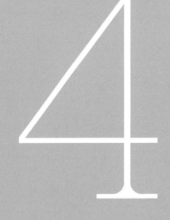

Be realistic

This may be slightly reiterating what I've spoken about at length regarding quick fixes, but I do feel it warrants another mention. One salad doesn't make you lose weight, while one bad meal doesn't make you put on weight.

It's here where I remind you that, as stated at the beginning of this section, slow and gradual change is undoubtedly going to provide you with the most sustainable and long-lasting results. Don't feel disheartened or beat yourself up because you see no instant visual change.

This book is about creating the happiest and healthiest version of you, both inside and out, and so the internal changes should be celebrated just as much as the external.

What I want
this book to
give to you:
The Promise

- A motivational tool to help you break free from fad diets and establish a year-round healthy body and mind.

- A no-nonsense guide to nutrition, explaining why I make the choices I do, with research-based evidence to accompany my decisions.

- A sustainable, balanced approach to nutrition, whereby calorie or macro counting is ditched for more intuitive eating.

- A flexible guide to how to build the perfect plates. I will give you examples for all situations, where I show you how and why I build my plates the way I do.

- An alternative to 'diets', whereby you focus on short- and long-term goals, both physically and mentally, that don't involve you stepping on the scales.

NUTRITION

Macronutrients: what are they and why do we need them?

You've often heard the word macronutrients or macros thrown around; perhaps like me, you've wondered what each of these individual food groups actually brought to the body and why we need them. What I intend to do is provide you with recipes that are nutrient dense, giving you a balanced intake of a wide variety of both macro- and micronutrients to optimise your health. I've touched on each of the macronutrients and explained their role within the body, as well as the value of all-important micronutrients. There are more qualified people and other books that go into much more detail. While I don't want to bog you down with nutritional dogma, I feel that understanding basic nutrition is essential to gaining control over your own eating. This will help you make your own choices about your diet, while also ensuring that you don't become deficient in any vital nutrients.

With the plate examples in this book, I aim to show you practical examples of exactly how I incorporate a balance of these important foods into my diet, so that it doesn't feel as though you're reading a science book! I'm a very visual person, so for me it is important to see how you actually put together a meal with both taste and nutrient density high on the agenda.

Proteins, fats and carbohydrates: what are they and why do we need them?

Protein

Protein is one of the three macronutrients that the body needs in order to function optimally. Protein is so important in our diet due to the abundance of roles that it performs within our bodies. Proteins make up the enzymes that power chemical reactions, they also make up the haemoglobin that transports oxygen in the blood and are the structural components of things like skin, hair, nails, tendons and ligaments. So it's quite important that we consume enough to support these basic bodily functions!

Protein is made up of building blocks called amino acids, and there are 21 types of amino acids. Of these, nine cannot be produced by the body and therefore must be derived from the food that we eat. These are therefore described as essential amino acids.

The protein that we eat can be divided into two main sources within the diet: animal proteins and plant proteins. Animal proteins, such as meat and fish, are examples of complete proteins because they contain all nine essential amino acids. Some plant proteins are complete proteins, too, such as quinoa, but most often plant-based proteins such as grains and legumes are missing one or more essential amino acids. However, by combining complementary plant-based proteins they become complete, such as combining rice with beans or hummus with wholegrain pitta bread.

Understanding that protein is essential to optimal bodily function, and isn't just for body builders, is one of the best lessons I learnt while transforming my diet. Personally, I wasn't eating enough protein, and so understanding that on average we need to consume roughly 0.8-1.5g of protein per kilogram of body weight was a useful figure to demonstrate how much I needed to be eating. If this is a little complicated for you, try just aiming for a fist full of protein with every main meal, whether that be a chicken breast, some salmon or lentils; ensuring you have a source of good-quality protein at each meal will help you to meet your daily required intake.

Variety is my best advice with all foods, and this can certainly be said for protein consumption. Eating a wide variety of sources of protein will ensure that you're also taking on a multitude of vitamins and minerals that can also be found in proteins, such as iron in red meat and omega-3s in oily fish.

Lastly, protein is believed to be the most satiating of the macronutrients, which means that it will keep you fuller for longer – yet another reason to ensure that you are eating enough of it!

Carbohydrates

Carbohydrates make up another third of the macronutrients, and are of equal importance to both proteins and fats. Carbohydrates are responsible for providing the body with energy via glycolysis. We often hear of carbohydrates categorised into two groups – complex carbohydrates and simple carbohydrates – but many people feel that this oversimplifies them, giving simple carbohydrates a bad name. For example, apples are a simple carbohydrate, however their nutritional profile is far greater than that of something like simple white sugar, and so calling them a simple carbohydrate is, to a certain extent, demonising a worthwhile ingredient in your diet. For this reason, many practitioners now use something called the glycemic load (GL), which is a development of the glycemic index – a scale that determines how quickly carbohydrate-based foods are absorbed and have an effect on blood glucose levels, considering the portion of food consumed. Without overcomplicating things, foods with a low glycemic load provide a slow release of energy, while foods with a high glycemic load provide a quicker release of energy into the blood stream. There are also other factors worth considering, such as fibre, sugar, protein and fat content found in the carbohydrate.

While I'm not trying to overwhelm you with information, it's good to understand the food you are putting into your body, and what happens when you eat it. The most important thing to take home here is that both high- and low-GL foods are useful in the diet, and neither should be restricted or feared; but harnessing the ability to select slower-releasing carbohydrates for prolonged energy and satiation may be preferable in many circumstances, and it is certainly something that I tend to stick to the majority of the time.

To sum up, try to go for healthier carbohydrates which come from unprocessed or minimally processed whole grains, vegetables, fruits and pulses and limit the unhealthier forms of carbohydrates, such as sugary fizzy drinks, white bread and sweets, as the sugar in these is very accessible to the body.

Fats

The last of the three macronutrients is fats. Fats have often had a bad reputation over the years, but for optimal health they should never be neglected from the diet.

Fats are generally broken down into three categories. The first is saturated fats, which are usually found in animal sources such as meat, butter and cheese, but can also be found in plant-based sources such as coconut oil. Saturated fats are solid at room temperature.

Unsaturated fats are the second grouping of fats, and are mostly found in plant sources. They are liquid at room temperature, and can be further categorised into two types – mono- and polyunsaturated fats. Mono- and polyunsaturated fats are the fats generally considered to be 'healthy fats'. Mono-unsaturated fats include things like olive oil, nuts and some fish oils. Examples of poly-unsaturated fats include things like walnuts, chia seeds and sunflower seeds.

The final type of fat found in our diet is trans fats. Trans fats do occur naturally in very small quantities but artificial trans fats are something that should be avoided on the whole. Artificial trans fats are man-made fats produced by hydrogenation, a chemical process that alters the structure of a polyunsaturated fat, and overconsumption of these types of fats has been linked with numerous negative health outcomes. A lot of work has been done by food manufacturers to reduce/remove trans fats from their food, but they do still exist. The best way to spot them is to look for partially hydrogenated fats or vegetable oils on an ingredients list.

So now we know which fats are beneficial to our diets and which we need to ditch, it's also important to understand the role that fats play within the body. Fatty acids we consume through food help contribute towards an array of bodily functions, from hormone regulation and assisting vitamin absorption to aiding growth and development. Omega-3 fatty acids are fats that appear regularly in my diet, and fall into the essential fatty acids category, meaning that the body does not produce them and so they have to be derived from our food. They can be found in foods such as oily fish, nuts and seeds.

My go-to fats are salmon, coconut oil, avocado, full-fat yoghurt, olive oil and nuts and seeds such as almonds and pumpkin seeds. I personally prefer to cook with coconut oil, which is very high in saturated fat and therefore should be consumed in moderation, so feel free to swap coconut oil for healthy polyunsaturated and monosaturated oils such as rapeseed and olive oil to ensure a balanced and healthy fat intake. However, it's best to stick to coconut oil for the baking recipes in this book as it's harder to successfully substitute in these recipes.

While it is important to understand the benefits of fats, it is also worth mentioning that they are almost twice as energy dense as carbohydrates and proteins, with 9kcals per gram of fat. This shouldn't alarm you, but sometimes it's necessary to exercise more portion control when eating foods rich in fats.

Micronutrients: what are they and why do we need them?

Despite being described as micro, micronutrients are of no less importance to our body than the macronutrients – it's just we need them in smaller quantities. These essential vitamins and minerals such as iron, zinc and B vitamins help contribute towards a whole host of functions within the body, however with a poor diet, it is easy to become deficient in them. Ensuring that you eat a wide variety of protein sources such as oily fish, wholegrains, pulses, vegetables, fruits and, on occasion, red meat, will help to avoid any such deficiency. When it comes to micronutrients, the phrase 'eat the rainbow' springs to mind, and this is certainly an easy way to remind yourself to incorporate a variety of colourful nutrient-rich foods into your diet.

Dietary fibre: what is it and why do we need it?

Dietary fibre is often overlooked when discussing nutrient intake, but it is of utmost importance in many bodily functions. Understanding what it is and what foods you can get it from will help to ensure that you are eating enough fibrous foods to keep your bowels regular and to help keep your blood sugar levels stable, through slowing down the release of sugars from digested food into the bloodstream.

There are two types of dietary fibre – soluble and insoluble. Soluble fibre dissolves in water to become viscous. It promotes the release of fatty substances such as cholesterol, and also helps to regulate the body's use of sugars. Soluble fibre can be found in foods such as legumes, oats, some fruits such as avocados, ripe bananas and plums, some vegetables such as broccoli, and sweet potato, flaxseeds and nuts such as almonds.

Insoluble fibre doesn't dissolve in water, but adds bulk and softness to stools, therefore promoting bowel regularity. Insoluble fibre can be found in foods such as whole grains, peas, nuts and seeds, cauliflower and the skin of fruits such as kiwis and tomatoes.

A diet naturally high in fibre also improves gastrointestinal health, has been shown to reduce the risk of developing conditions such as heart disease, diabetes and cancer, increase satiety and reduce blood pressure. So if all of this seems a little intense, just see it as another important reason to eat your wholegrains and greens!

Sugar: the facts

Sugar appears to be the current hot topic of discussion, so I wanted to discuss it briefly to alleviate any confusion regarding intake.

'Sugars' are carbohydrates, which provide fuel (energy) for the body. The term 'sugars' covers a range of different types of sugar structures, from fructose, sucrose, glucose and lactose to maltose and more. These occur naturally in foods such as fruits, vegetables and dairy products, but are also added to a wide range of foods and drinks.

While it's important to remember that, yes, the body does need carbohydrates as a source of energy, the sugars found in many processed foods hold very little, if any, nutritional value – which therefore begs the question, why do we need them? When any carbohydrate is ingested, it is broken down into monosaccharides, or simple sugars, before being absorbed by our bodies. This is irrespective of whether the food source is a simple sugar cube or a sweet potato. The only difference between these two, once ingested, is that the 'healthier' sweet potato is nutrient dense and packed full of fibre and micronutrients. It is also digested and absorbed much more slowly than the nutrient-free sugar cube, which is delivered into the bloodstream very quickly.

Once broken down and absorbed, sugars go to the liver to fill our energy stores, before entering the bloodstream and then passing into other cells of the body. At this point, the hormone insulin is released to control this sugar load.

The reason why we must be mindful of the source of our carbohydrates (and why I tend to opt for nutrient-dense, high-fibre carbohydrates such as a sweet potato) is that, when the diet consists of simple sugars and refined carbohydrates, you can experience sharp elevations in blood sugar levels. This is often followed by crashes, resulting in a vicious cycle of energy highs and lows. If overconsumed, there is also the possibility of elevation in blood triglyceride levels, bad cholesterol and increased insulin resistance. Carbohydrates that are digested and absorbed slowly, such as whole grains, fruits and vegetables, can help to control insulin response. This means more even energy levels, but most importantly, a whole host of added nutrient benefits such as increased vitamin, mineral and fibre intake and enhanced satiety, too.

The NHS advises that we reserve only 5% of our total daily caloric intake for added sugars, which equates to around 30g of sugar.

My own approach? I don't think we should fear sugar: it isn't the devil, but equally if overconsumed it can cause weight gain and have serious health implications. My approach to eating means that I try to obtain the majority of my diet from single ingredient, natural foods, and therefore the majority of my recipes contain little, if any, refined sugars.

Although they contain some sugars in the form of maple or date syrup, the snacks, sweets and treats recipes mean that you're not totally denying yourself that sweet, delicious flavour that we all love. But by making these from scratch, not only are they often paired with a nutrient-dense complex carbohydrate or fibre source to help slow the release of sugars into the bloodstream, but you also know each ingredient you are putting into your body. This approach is far better than relying on shop-bought equivalents, which can have a perplexing list of ingredients.

RECIPES

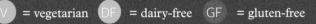

V = vegetarian   DF = dairy-free   GF = gluten-free

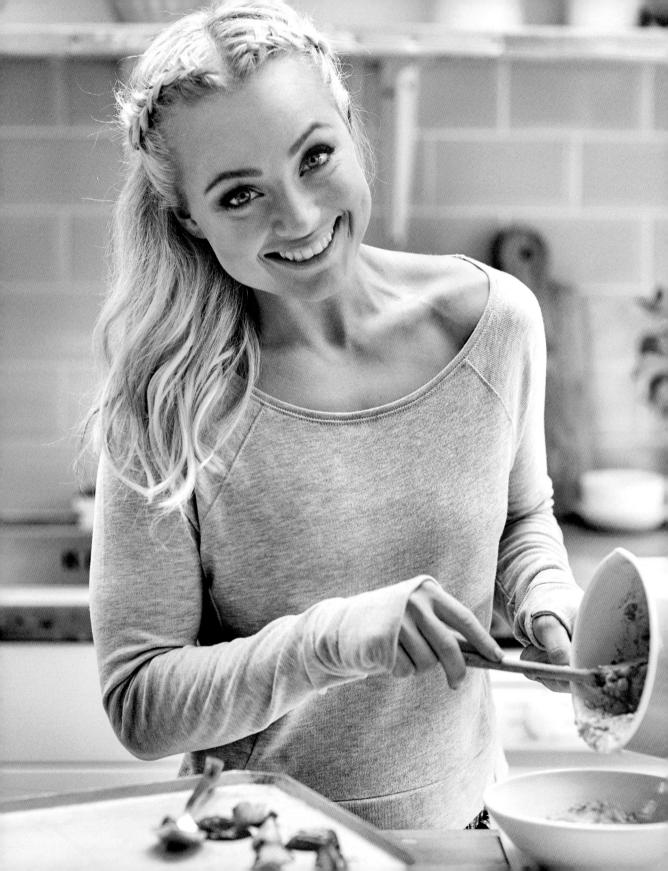

BREAKFAST

Maple Syrup French Toast with Greek Yoghurt and Homemade Strawberry Chia Jam

V

The ultimate indulgent weekend breakfast. Need I say more...?

2 tbsp chia seeds
250g strawberries, hulled
2 tbsp maple syrup
1 free-range egg
50ml unsweetened almond milk
½ tsp ground cinnamon
½ tsp coconut oil
4 slices of sourdough or rye bread
2 tbsp Greek yoghurt

SERVES 2

Begin by grinding the chia seeds in a small food processor for a few minutes until fine. Add the strawberries and 1 tablespoon of the maple syrup and blitz for a further minute.

Place a saucepan over a medium heat, add the strawberry mixture and cook for 5–7 minutes, until thickened and jammy, stirring often. Pour into a bowl and leave to cool.

Meanwhile, crack the egg into a large shallow bowl. Add the almond milk, cinnamon and remaining tablespoon of maple syrup and whisk.

Heat the coconut oil in a large non-stick frying pan over a medium-high heat until melted.

Coat each slice of bread on both sides in the egg mixture, then add to the pan; you may need to do this in batches. Cook for 1 minute on each side until golden and crispy, and serve topped with a spoonful of Greek yoghurt and the strawberry chia jam.

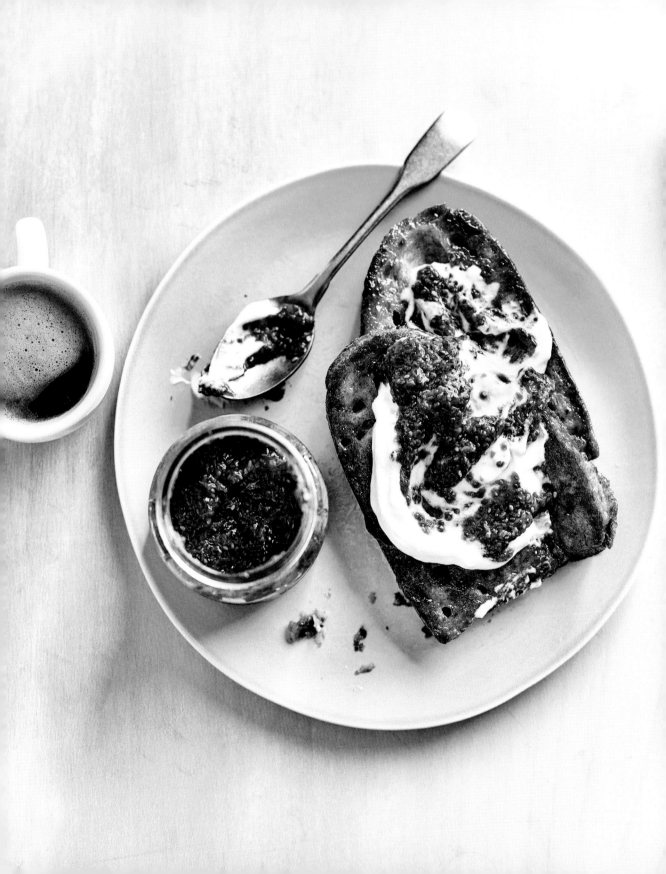

Crispy Courgette Fritters with Smoked Salmon

DF **GF**

Packed full of goodness, these courgette fritters couldn't be simpler to make, and are the perfect way to start your day. Paired with smoked salmon – a top-quality source of protein and fat – this dish is great brain fuel for those busy days.

50g rolled oats
1 free-range egg
2 large firm courgettes, cut into 5cm batons
2 tbsp coconut oil
100g smoked salmon
100g fresh spinach, finely chopped
extra virgin olive oil, for drizzling
½ lemon, cut into wedges
sea salt and freshly ground black pepper

SERVES 2

Begin by blitzing the oats in a food processor to a flour-like consistency, then tip onto a plate.

Crack the egg into a small bowl, whisk and set aside.

Dip each courgette baton in the whisked egg, then roll in the oat flour to lightly coat.

Heat the coconut oil in a large wok or frying pan over a medium-high heat until melted.

Carefully add the coated batons and fry until golden on all sides and cooked through; you may need to do this in batches.

Remove from the pan with a slotted spatula and serve with the smoked salmon and chopped spinach. Season with a little salt and black pepper, drizzle with olive oil and serve with lemon wedges for squeezing over.

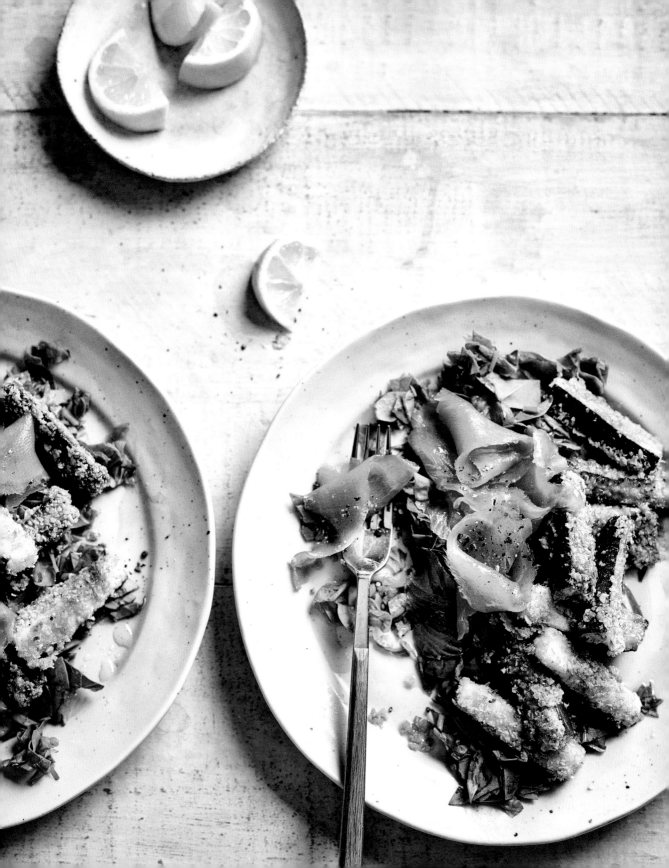

Mushroom, Spinach and Feta Omelette

GF V

Quick, easy, simple and delicious, what's not to love about omelettes? Spinach gives a boost of vitamin K for strong bones, while eggs are a super-healthy, protein-packed way to start the day.

1 tsp coconut oil
5–6 chestnut mushrooms, thinly sliced
a small handful of fresh spinach
3 free-range eggs
1 tbsp unsweetened almond milk
30g feta, crumbled
a pinch of chilli flakes
sea salt and freshly ground black pepper

SERVES 1

Heat the coconut oil in a large non-stick frying pan over a medium-high heat until melted.

Add the mushrooms, season with salt and pepper and fry for 7–10 minutes until golden, stirring occasionally.

Add the spinach for the final minute to wilt, then tip the vegetables onto a plate and set aside.

Crack the eggs into a large bowl and whisk until fully combined. Add the milk and a pinch of salt and pepper and whisk for a further few seconds.

Return the pan to a medium-low heat, pour in the egg mixture and leave to cook for a few minutes until the base begins to set.

Evenly scatter over the mushrooms, spinach, feta and chilli flakes. Once the top of the omelette has almost set, fold to seal, then serve.

Smoked Salmon and Dill Omelette with Spiced Greek Yoghurt

Salmon and dill is a classic flavour combination - adding creamy Greek yoghurt mixed with paprika provides a spiced twist.

3 free-range eggs
1 tbsp unsweetened almond milk
½ lemon, zested and cut into wedges
1 tsp coconut oil
50g smoked salmon, thinly sliced
a few sprigs of fresh dill, chopped
50g Greek yoghurt
½ tsp smoked paprika
sea salt and freshly ground black
    pepper

SERVES 1

Crack the eggs into a large bowl and whisk until fully combined. Add the milk, lemon zest and a pinch of salt and pepper and whisk for a further few seconds.

Heat the coconut oil in a large non-stick frying pan over a medium-low heat until melted. Pour in the egg mixture and leave to cook for a few minutes until the base begins to set.

Evenly scatter over the smoked salmon and dill.

While the omelette cooks, mix the Greek yoghurt with the smoked paprika and a pinch of salt and black pepper.

Once the top of the omelette has almost set, fold to seal and serve topped with the spiced Greek yoghurt and lemon wedges for squeezing over.

Spicy Baked Butter Beans on Toast

(DF) (V)

Who doesn't love beans on toast? With an added kick of paprika, this version of the classic breakfast will become a firm favourite.

1 tsp coconut oil
1 small onion, peeled, halved and thinly sliced
½ tsp smoked paprika
400g tinned chopped tomatoes
400g tinned butter beans, drained
2 thick slices of sourdough bread
a couple of sprigs of fresh parsley, leaves chopped
sea salt and freshly ground black pepper

SERVES 2

Heat the coconut oil in a medium saucepan over a medium-low heat until melted.

Add the onion, paprika and a little salt and pepper. Stir to coat, then cover and cook for 5–7 minutes until softened, stirring occasionally.

Add the chopped tomatoes and butter beans, bring to the boil, then reduce the heat to low and simmer for around 15 minutes until cooked through, stirring occasionally.

Toast the sourdough, serve topped with a large spoonful of the butter beans and sprinkle with the parsley.

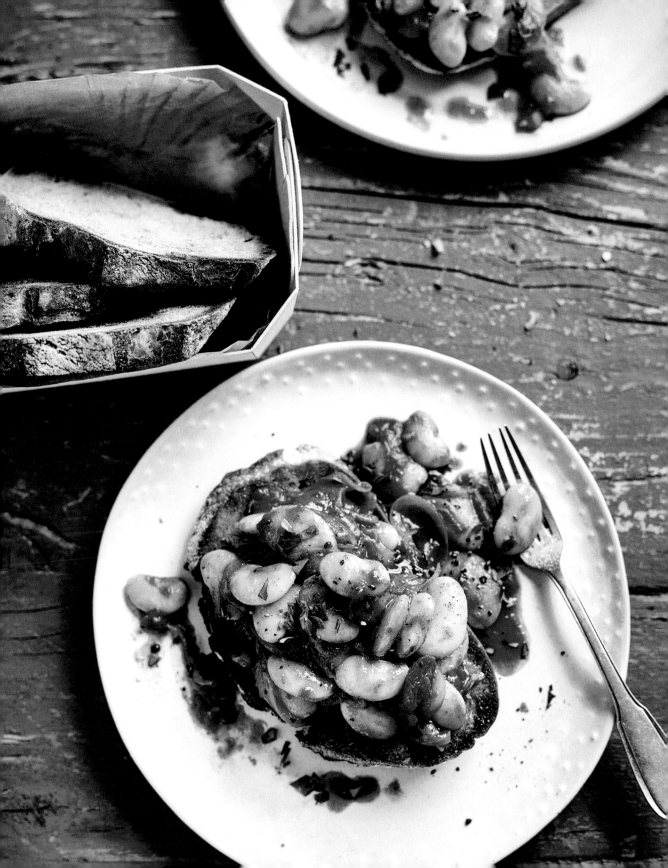

Poached Eggs with Broccoli, Feta, Chilli and Garlic

GF V

Simple, spicy, seriously good. Nothing fancy here, just some awesome flavours to awaken your taste buds with a bang!

20g flaked almonds

1 tsp coconut oil

200g Tenderstem broccoli, trimmed

1 small garlic clove, peeled and finely chopped

1 tbsp cider vinegar

2 free-range eggs

1 small red chilli, deseeded and thinly sliced

30g feta, crumbled

sea salt and freshly ground black pepper

SERVES 1

Toast the almonds in a dry frying pan over a medium-high heat until lightly golden, shaking the pan often. Tip onto a plate and return the pan to the heat.

Add the coconut oil. Once melted, add the broccoli and fry for 7–10 minutes, turning often, adding the garlic for the final minute.

Meanwhile, fill a saucepan three-quarters full with water, bring to the boil and add the cider vinegar.

Reduce the heat to medium-low. Once gently simmering, swiftly crack in each egg and poach for 3–4 minutes.

Remove the broccoli to a plate and top with the chilli, flaked almonds and crumbled feta.

Remove the eggs from the pan with a slotted spoon, place on top of the broccoli, season with a little salt and pepper and serve.

Fried Eggs with Quinoa, Kale, Pomegranate and Pumpkin Seeds

(GF) (DF) (V)

Packed full of protein and fibre, this breakfast offers a slow release of energy to keep you fuelled during those busy days!

100g quinoa, rinsed
2 tsp coconut oil
200g kale, large stems removed
2 tbsp pumpkin seeds
½ tsp ground cumin
4 free-range eggs
2 tbsp pomegranate seeds
sea salt and freshly ground black
     pepper

SERVES 2

Put the quinoa into a saucepan, cover with cold salted water and place over a medium heat. Bring to the boil, reduce the heat to low and simmer for 15 minutes until cooked through, adding extra water if needed. Drain and set aside.

While the quinoa is cooking, massage 1 teaspoon of the coconut oil into the kale until completely coated. Season with a little salt and pepper.

Toast the pumpkin seeds in a large dry frying pan over a medium heat for a few minutes until lightly toasted, shaking the pan often. Tip onto a plate and return the frying pan to a medium heat. Add the kale to the pan with ¼ teaspoon of the cumin and fry until the kale is softened, stirring often. Tip into a mixing bowl.

Return the frying pan to the heat and add the remaining teaspoon of coconut oil. Once melted, crack in each egg; you may need to do this in batches.

Stir the remaining ¼ teaspoon cumin into the quinoa with most of the pomegranate seeds. Add to the kale, stir to combine, divide between two plates and top with the fried eggs. Sprinkle with the toasted pumpkin seeds and the remaining pomegranate seeds.

Dippy Eggs with Roasted Parsnip Soldiers

A grown-up twist on a childhood breakfast favourite, this is the perfect way to start a weekend or lazy day.

1 tsp coconut oil
500g parsnips, peeled and cut into
    5cm batons
½ tsp ground cumin
4 free-range eggs
sea salt

SERVES 2

Preheat the oven to 200°C/400°F/Gas Mark 6. Put the coconut oil into a roasting tray and place in the oven to melt.

Once the coconut oil has melted, remove the tray from the oven, tip in the parsnips and toss to coat. Season with cumin and salt and roast in the oven for 40 minutes, tossing halfway through.

Just before the parsnips are cooked, bring a saucepan of salted water to the boil. Carefully lower in the eggs, reduce the heat to medium and simmer for 5 minutes.

Drain the eggs, place in egg cups and use a knife to remove the top of each egg. Serve with the roasted parsnips for dipping.

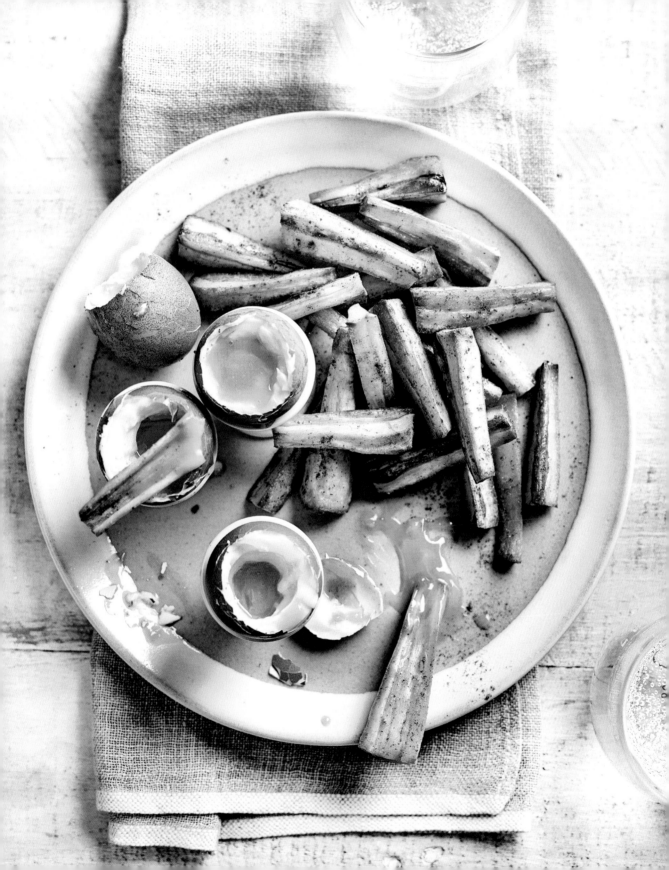

Full English Breakfast Frittata

 DF GF

A one-pan wonder that packs your favourite 'fry-up' ingredients into a healthier and super-simple take on the classic dish.

2 tsp coconut oil

2 venison sausages

2–3 lean bacon medallions

4 free-range eggs

a handful of fresh chives, chopped

8 button mushrooms, halved

8 cherry tomatoes, halved

sea salt and freshly ground black pepper

SERVES 2

Preheat the grill to medium.

Heat 1 teaspoon of the coconut oil in a large non-stick ovenproof pan over a medium heat until melted. Add the sausages and cook for 5–7 minutes, until lightly browned.

Add the bacon and cook with the sausages, until both are cooked through, turning halfway.

Tip onto a plate and pat with kitchen paper to remove any excess fat. Leave to cool, then cut into chunks.

Crack the eggs into a bowl and whisk until fully combined. Season well with salt and pepper, then add the chives and whisk again.

Return the pan to a medium heat, heat the remaining teaspooon of coconut oil until melted and add the mushrooms. Cook for 5–7 minutes until nicely golden, then add the tomatoes and cook for a further 2 minutes.

Pour in the egg mixture. Once starting to set, add the bacon and sausages and place the pan under the grill for 2–5 minutes until set and cooked through.

Chorizo and Feta Mini Egg Muffins

GF

Perfect pre-prepared yumminess, these store well in the fridge so are another great idea for on-the-go food for busy mornings.

coconut oil, for greasing
4 free-range eggs
50g feta, crumbled
50g fresh spinach, finely chopped
50g dry cured chorizo, roughly
    chopped
sea salt and freshly ground black
    pepper

MAKES 6

Preheat the oven to 180°C/350°F/Gas Mark 4 and grease six wells of a muffin tin with coconut oil.

Crack the eggs into a bowl and whisk until fully combined. Add the feta, spinach and chorizo and season to taste.

Divide the mixture between the six greased wells and cook in the preheated oven for 10–15 minutes or until golden.

Leave to cool for a few minutes before serving. The muffins can be stored in an airtight container in the fridge for 2 days.

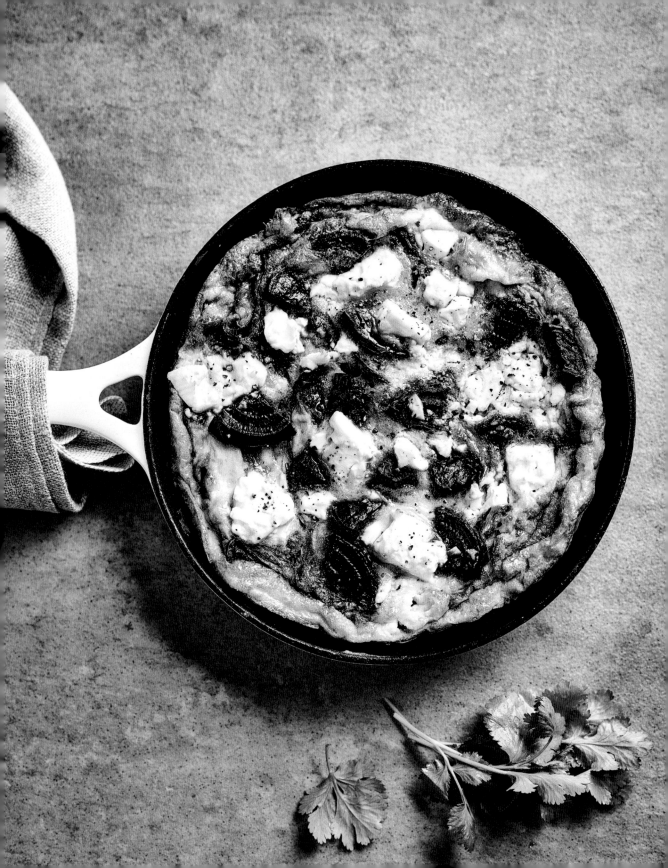

Beetroot and Feta Frittata

GF **V**

Packed full of colour and flavour, this is the perfect recipe for cooking once and eating twice – pop it into a sealable container to take half to work or store it in the fridge for tomorrow's breakfast!

1½ tbsp coconut oil
2 beetroots, peeled, trimmed and roughly chopped
6 free-range eggs
1 red onion, peeled, halved and finely sliced
100g feta, crumbled
a few sprigs of fresh coriander, leaves chopped
sea salt and freshly ground black pepper

SERVES 2

Preheat the oven to 200°C/400°F/Gas Mark 6.

Put 1 tablespoon of the coconut oil into a small roasting tray and place in the oven to melt.

Once the coconut oil has melted, remove the tray from the oven, tip in the chopped beetroot and toss to coat.

Season with salt and pepper and roast in the hot oven for 40 minutes or until softened, tossing halfway through. Remove from the oven and set aside.

Preheat the grill to high.

Crack the eggs into a bowl with a pinch of salt and pepper and whisk until fully combined.

Heat the remaining ½ tablespoon of coconut oil in a large non-stick ovenproof pan over a medium heat. Add the red onion and fry for 5–7 minutes, until soft.

Add the beetroot and feta and pour in the egg mixture. Once starting to set, place the pan under the grill for a few minutes until set, then serve scattered with the coriander.

Smoked Mackerel with Wilted Spinach and Avocado

(GF)

Beginning your day with a rich source of omega-3 fatty acids helps to keep your heart healthy. Paired with some fresh avocado, this combination is both nutritious and delicious.

200g smoked mackerel, skin removed

1 tbsp Greek yoghurt

1 lemon, ½ juiced, ½ cut into wedges

a pinch of chilli flakes

½ tsp coconut oil

1 garlic clove, peeled and minced

200g fresh spinach

1 ripe avocado, peeled, stoned and sliced

sea salt and freshly ground black pepper

SERVES 2

Put the mackerel into a large mixing bowl and season with a little salt and pepper.

Add the Greek yoghurt, lemon juice and chilli flakes and mash with a fork until fully combined.

Heat the coconut oil in a large frying pan over a medium heat until melted. Add the garlic and cook for 30 seconds before adding the spinach in batches until wilted, stirring often.

Season with a little salt and pepper and serve with the sliced avocado, mackerel mixture and lemon wedges for squeezing over.

Spicy Smoked Mackerel on Toast

Another tasty combination of healthy fats, protein and carbohydrates to ensure that you're fuelled the right way first thing in the morning.

1 tbsp Greek yoghurt
1 tsp harissa paste
½ lemon, juiced
200g smoked mackerel, skin removed
2 thick slices of sourdough bread
2 small handfuls of rocket
sea salt and freshly ground black
   pepper

SERVES 2

Put the yoghurt, harissa and lemon juice into a bowl with a pinch of salt and pepper and stir to combine.

Flake in the mackerel and mix and mash with a fork until combined.

Toast the bread, top with the rocket and the mackerel mixture and serve.

Ultimate Breakfast Wrap with Homemade Chunky Salsa

This wrap brings together some of my favourite foods into one recipe and, paired with some homemade spicy salsa, it is an impressive way to start the day.

2 tsp extra virgin olive oil
½ small red onion, peeled and finely chopped
10 cherry tomatoes, halved
a pinch of chilli flakes
a squeeze of lemon juice
a small handful of fresh coriander, leaves roughly chopped
3 free-range eggs
2 small wholemeal wraps
60g dry cured chorizo, cut into chunks
6 chestnut mushrooms, thinly sliced
100g fresh spinach
30g feta, crumbled
sea salt and freshly ground black pepper

SERVES 2

Preheat the oven to 150°C/300°F/Gas Mark 2.

Begin by making the salsa. Heat 1 teaspoon of the olive oil in a small saucepan over a medium-low heat. Add the onion and cook for 5–7 minutes until softened, stirring occasionally.

Add the tomatoes and chilli flakes and cook for a further 3 minutes, or until the tomatoes have softened.

Add the lemon juice, coriander and remaining teaspoon of the olive oil, season to taste and set aside.

Crack the eggs into a bowl and whisk until fully combined. Place the wraps in the oven to warm through.

Place a frying pan over a medium-high heat and add the chorizo. Cook until it starts to release its oil, then add the mushrooms and cook for a few minutes until golden, stirring occasionally.

Add the spinach and cook until it is starting to wilt. Pour in the egg mixture and stir slowly and continuously to scramble.

When the eggs are almost cooked, stir in the feta. Divide the egg scramble between the two wraps, top with the homemade chunky salsa, then fold up and serve.

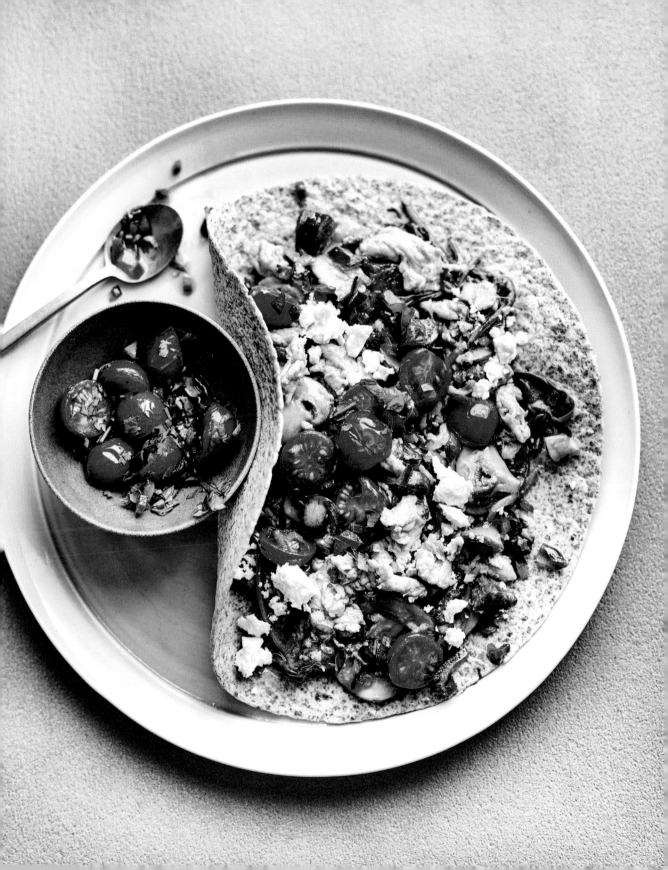

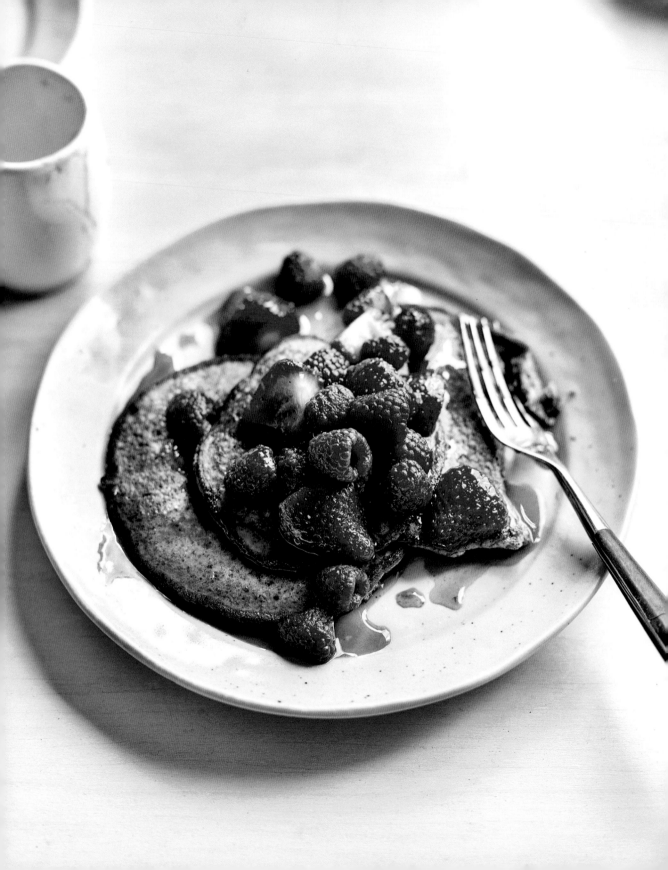

Four-ingredient Banana Pancakes with Warm Berry Compote

DF GF V

Sweet and deliciously light, these pancakes are the ultimate morning treat to satisfy any sweet tooth.

1 large ripe banana, peeled
2 free-range eggs, plus 1 egg white
2 tbsp milled flaxseed
½ tsp ground cinnamon
2 tsp coconut oil
1 tsp honey
50g raspberries
50g strawberries, hulled and chopped

SERVES 1

Mash the banana in a bowl with a fork until smooth, then add the eggs and egg white and whisk again until completely combined.

Add the flaxseed and cinnamon and whisk again.

Heat 1 teaspoon of the coconut oil in a large non-stick frying pan until melted, then gradually pour in a quarter of the mixture. Repeat with the remaining mixture until you have three pancakes; you may have to do this in batches.

When bubbles begin to appear on the surface of the pancakes, flip them over, then cook until golden and cooked through.

Meanwhile, melt the remaining 1 teaspoon of coconut oil in a saucepan over a medium-low heat. Once melted, add the honey and berries and cook for 2 minutes, until warmed through, then serve on top of the pancakes.

Coconut and Fig Overnight Chia Pudding

GF V

Packed full of plant-based protein, the use of chia seeds make this pudding a nutritious way to start your day.

3 tbsp chia seeds
1 tsp honey
2 tbsp Greek yoghurt
250ml tinned coconut milk
10g flaked almonds
1 ripe fig, quartered

SERVES 1

Put the chia seeds, honey and yoghurt into a bowl. Add most of the coconut milk and stir until fully combined. Cover and place in the fridge overnight.

In the morning, toast the almonds in a small dry pan over a medium heat until lightly golden, shaking the pan often. Tip onto a plate.

Add the fig to the pan and heat until softened and gooey.

Loosen the pudding with a touch more coconut milk, if needed, then serve topped with the fig and almonds.

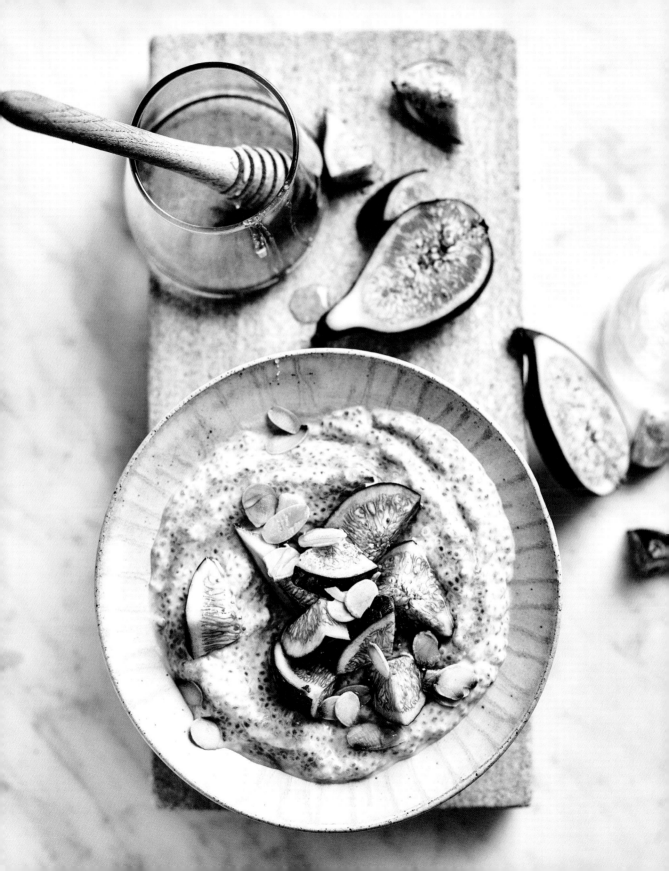

Greek Yoghurt with Warm Cinnamon-spiced Stewed Blueberry and Apple

Packed full of protein and berry sweetness, this quick-and-simple breakfast is one of my favourites to kick-start a busy day.

1 cooking apple, peeled, cored and
   chopped into 1cm chunks
½ tsp ground cinnamon
½ tsp vanilla extract
250g blueberries
1 tbsp sunflower seeds
1 tbsp pumpkin seeds
300g Greek yoghurt

SERVES 2

Put the apple into a medium saucepan with 3 tablespoons of water. Place over a medium heat and bring to the boil.

Reduce the heat to low, cover with a lid and simmer gently for 10–15 minutes, until softened.

Add the cinnamon, vanilla extract and blueberries and continue to simmer over a low heat until the blueberries are starting to soften but are still holding their shape.

Meanwhile, toast the seeds in a dry frying pan over a medium heat for a couple of minutes until lightly toasted, shaking the pan often.

Divide the yoghurt between two bowls, top with the stewed fruit and sprinkle over the toasted seeds.

Creamy Coconut Oats with Kiwi and Almond Butter

(DF) (GF) (V)

This is a winter-warmer indulgent treat to entice you out of bed on those dark mornings. Using the fruit's natural sweetness ensures a more nutritious breakfast than those sugar-laden cereals.

50g rolled oats
200ml unsweetened coconut milk or
    water, plus extra to loosen
50g desiccated coconut
1 kiwi, peeled and thinly sliced
1 tbsp almond butter

SERVES 1

Put the oats and coconut milk or water into a small saucepan over medium-low heat and gently simmer for a few minutes until thickened, stirring often, adding an extra splash of milk or water to loosen, if needed.

Stir in the desiccated coconut and serve topped with the sliced kiwi and almond butter.

Vanilla, Plum and Pistachio Power Oats

GF V

Porridge just got seriously good. This recipe feels indulgent yet light and is the perfect way to warm up on chilly mornings.

½ tsp coconut oil, for greasing
1 large ripe plum, halved, stoned and cut into thin wedges
50g rolled oats
200ml unsweetened almond milk or water
½ tsp ground cinnamon
½–1 scoop of vanilla whey protein
15g pistachio nuts, shelled
1 tsp honey

SERVES 1

Preheat the oven to 180°C/350°F/Gas Mark 4, line a small baking tray with foil and lightly grease with coconut oil.

Place the plum wedges on the baking tray and roast in the oven for 15 minutes or until softened, turning halfway through.

Put the oats into a small saucepan, add the almond milk or water and cinnamon and gently simmer for a few minutes, stirring often. Stir in the protein powder and continue to cook for a further minute or until thickened, adding an extra splash of milk or water to loosen if needed.

Roughly chop the pistachio nuts or place in a sandwich bag and bash with a rolling pin.

Serve the porridge topped with the roasted plum wedges and crushed pistachios and drizzle with the honey.

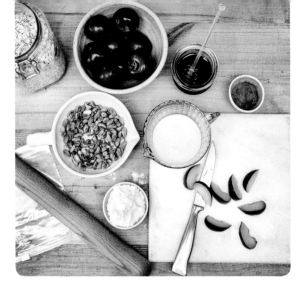

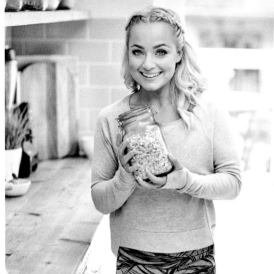

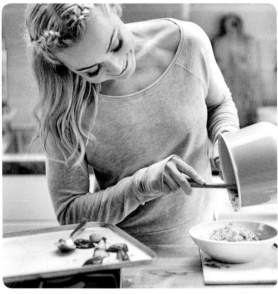

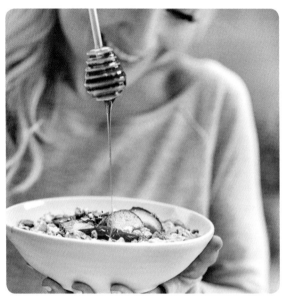

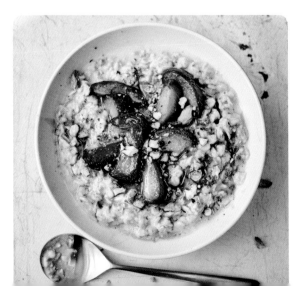

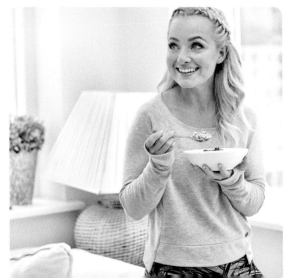

Overnight Oats Two Ways

Vanilla Overnight Oats with a Sweet Strawberry Sauce

I love this sauce. It's perfect for adding a sweet fruity twist to these simple creamy vanilla oats.

8 strawberries, hulled and quartered
½ orange, zested
½ tsp ground cinnamon
1 tsp honey
50g rolled oats
200ml unsweetened almond milk
½ tsp vanilla extract
2 tbsp chia seeds
1 tbsp dried cranberries
1 tbsp pumpkin seeds

SERVES 1

Put the strawberries, orange zest, cinnamon and honey into a bowl and mash to a pulp with a fork.

Cover the bowl with cling film and place in the fridge overnight.

In another bowl, mix together the oats, almond milk, vanilla extract, chia seeds, dried cranberries and pumpkin seeds. Cover and place in the fridge overnight.

In the morning, simply stir the oats and serve with the strawberry sauce.

Chocolate Orange Overnight Oats

A classic twist on a much-loved flavour combination that will satisfy a sweet tooth in the morning as well as keep you fuelled.

50g rolled oats
200ml unsweetened almond milk
1 large orange, zested and peeled
1 tbsp honey
1 tbsp cacao powder
cacao nibs (optional)

SERVES 1

Mix together the oats, almond milk, orange zest, honey and cacao powder until fully combined.

Slice the orange into thin rounds and line a jar or dish with these slices. Add the oat mixture to the jar or dish, then pop a lid on top or cover with foil and place in the fridge overnight.

In the morning, add the cacao nibs, if using, and serve.

Chocolate and Banana Protein Power Oats

GF **V**

Sweet, satiating and absolutely delicious. The ultimate post-workout yumminess, which delivers the perfect energy refuel for both mind and body.

1 ripe banana, peeled
50g rolled oats
200ml unsweetened almond milk or water
1 free-range egg white
1 tsp cacao powder
½–1 scoop of chocolate whey protein
20g 80% dark chocolate

SERVES 1

In a bowl, mash the banana with a fork until smooth.

Put the oats into a small saucepan, add the almond milk or water and egg white and whisk until combined.

Add the cacao powder and mashed banana, place over a medium-low heat and gently simmer for a few minutes, stirring often.

Stir in the protein powder and continue to cook for a further minute or until thickened, adding an extra splash of milk or water to loosen if needed.

Roughly chop the chocolate or place in a sandwich bag and bash with a rolling pin.

Serve the porridge topped with the dark chocolate.

Raspberry and Coconut Breakfast Loaf

(DF) (GF) (V)

Breakfast loaves are so great for grabbing on-the-go, and this deliciously sweet loaf is a firm favourite of mine in the morning. 'Bread' just got very interesting!

coconut oil, for greasing
175g almonds or ground almonds
25g desiccated coconut, plus extra to
    serve
1 lemon, zested
2 tsp baking powder
3 free-range eggs
5 tbsp honey, plus extra to serve
150g raspberries, plus extra to serve
sea salt

MAKES A 450G (1LB) LOAF

Preheat the oven to 180°C/350°F/Gas Mark 4. Grease and line a 450g (1lb) loaf tin.

Blitz the almonds in a food processor to a flour-like consistency (if you are using ground almonds, skip this step).

In a mixing bowl, mix together the ground almonds, desiccated coconut, lemon zest and baking powder with a pinch of sea salt.

In another bowl, whisk the eggs until fully combined, then add the honey.

Add the wet mixture to the dry mixture, then gently fold in the raspberries.

Carefully pour the mixture into the lined tin, gently pressing in the extra raspberries.

Bake in the hot oven for 50–60 minutes, until cooked through and a knife inserted comes out clean, covering with foil for the final 20 minutes.

Brush with honey and sprinkle with the extra desiccated coconut. Transfer to a wire rack to cool, then slice and serve.

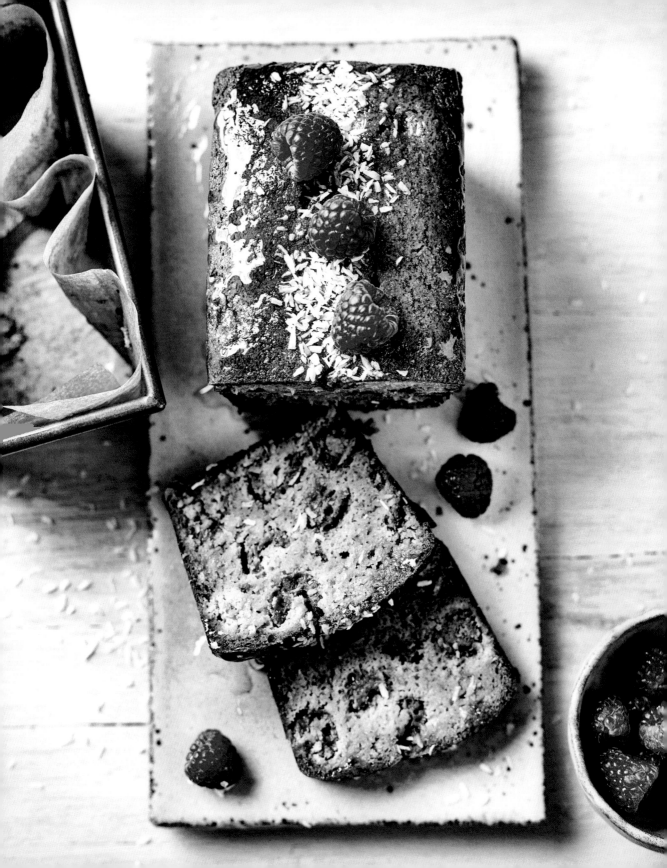

Blueberry and Avocado Breakfast Muffins

V

These are so moreish and the ultimate on-the-go breakfast treat. If you've got a busy week ahead, a batch of these will ensure that you don't find yourself going hungry in the morning.

250g spelt flour
2 tsp baking powder
½ tsp bicarbonate of soda
½ tsp sea salt
1 ripe avocado, peeled, halved and stoned
75g coconut sugar
2 free-range eggs
1 tsp vanilla extract
1 tbsp Greek yoghurt
65ml unsweetened almond milk
200g blueberries

MAKES 12

Preheat the oven to 180°C/350°F/Gas Mark 4 and line a muffin tin with 12 muffin cases.

In a mixing bowl, combine the spelt flour, baking powder, bicarbonate of soda and salt.

In a separate bowl, mash the avocado until smooth. Add the coconut sugar and mix until combined. Crack in the eggs, vanilla extract, yoghurt and almond milk and whisk until smooth.

Fold in the flour mixture bit by bit, then gently fold in the blueberries.

Divide the mixture evenly between the cases.

Bake in the hot oven for around 20 minutes, or until cooked through and a knife inserted comes out clean. Transfer to a wire rack to cool.

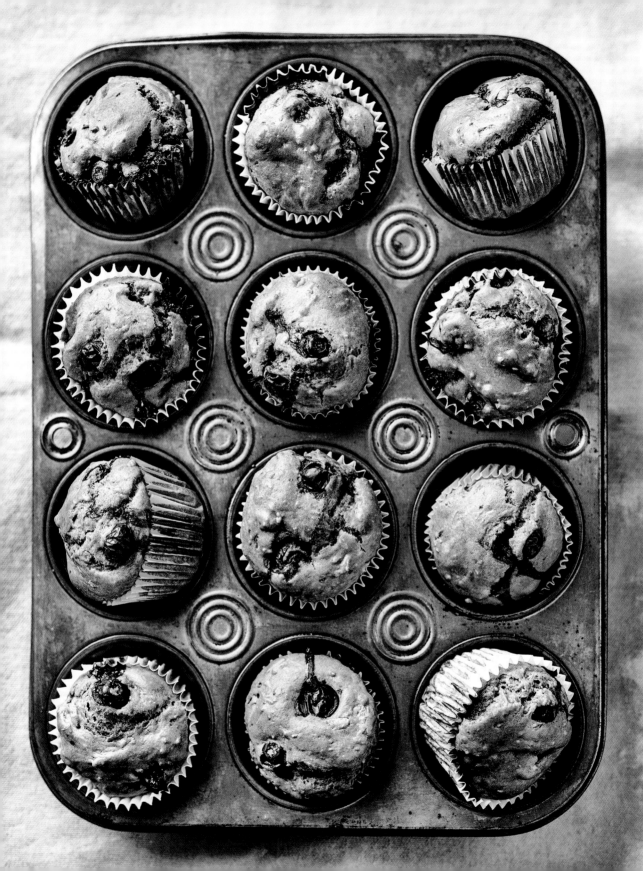

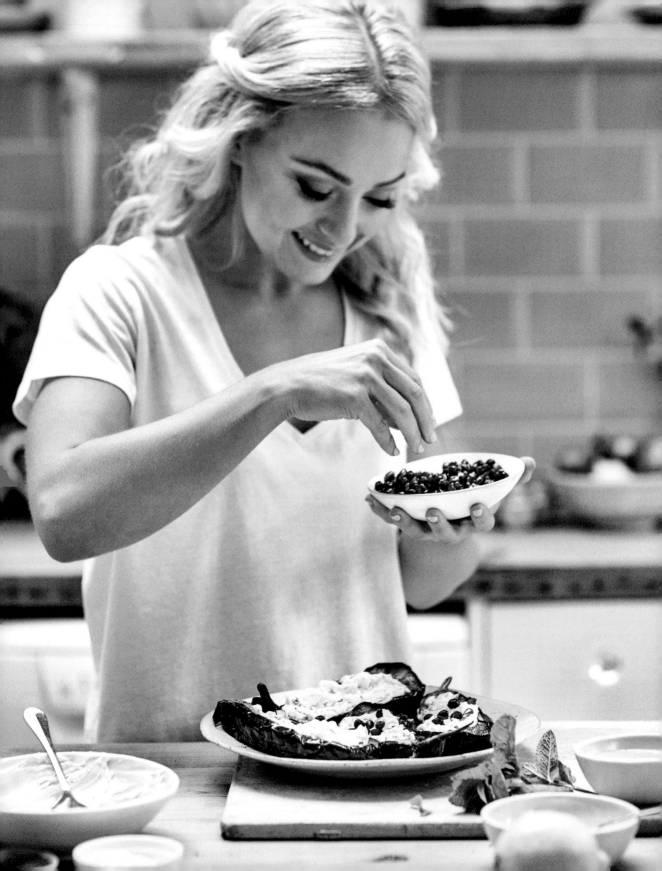

LUNCH

Salmon, Seeds, Avocado and Dill

(GF) (DF)

Simple, satisfying salmon is always a good idea for a packed lunch. Paired with avocado and seeds, this packs in healthy fats a-plenty.

2 salmon fillets
½ lemon, ½ sliced and ½ juiced
100g watercress
1 ripe avocado, peeled, halved, stoned
    and roughly chopped
2 free-range eggs
a few sprigs of fresh dill, chopped
1 tbsp pumpkin seeds
extra virgin olive oil, for drizzling
sea salt and freshly ground black
    pepper

SERVES 2

Preheat the oven to 200°C/400°F/Gas Mark 6.

Place each salmon fillet on a large piece of foil. Season well with a little salt and black pepper and add a slice of lemon to each fillet before wrapping tightly in the foil. Place on a baking tray and cook in the hot oven for about 12 minutes, or until cooked through.

Meanwhile, divide the watercress between two sealable containers. Add the avocado and squeeze over the lemon juice.

Place the eggs in a saucepan. Fill three-quarters full with water and bring to the boil. Reduce the heat to low and simmer for about 8 minutes. Drain and run the eggs under cold water for a few minutes before carefully removing the shells and slicing each egg into thick slices.

Once the salmon is cooked, gently break it into chunks, discarding the skin, and add it to the containers. Finally, add the sliced egg, sprinkle over the dill and pumpkin seeds, and finish with a pinch of black pepper. Drizzle with olive oil just before tucking in.

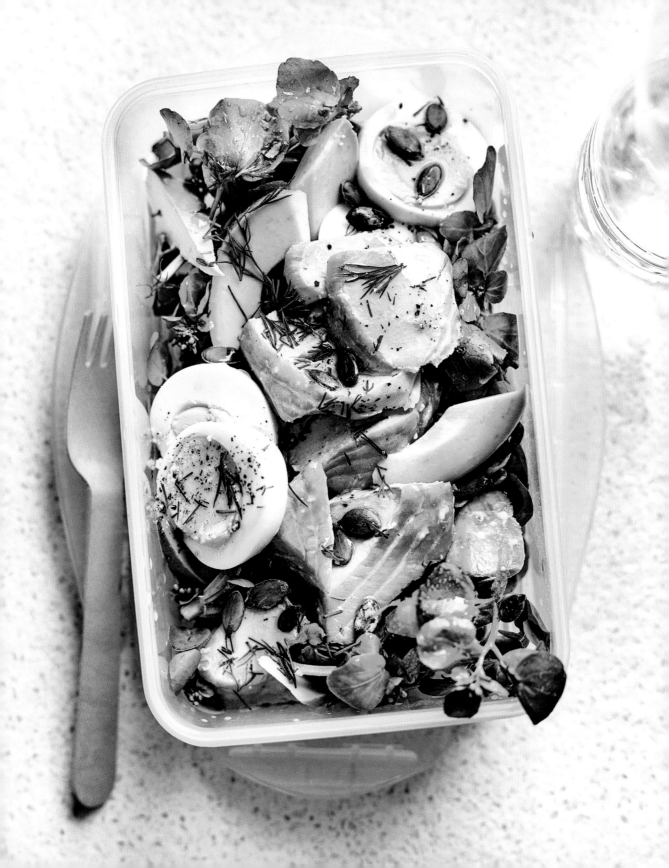

Steak and Balsamic Caramelised Red Onion Wrap

Feels naughty, tastes SO nice. Try it...

1 tbsp coconut oil

20g butter

1 large red onion, peeled, halved and finely sliced

1 shallot, peeled and finely chopped

1 tbsp balsamic vinegar

2 rump steaks, fat trimmed

2 wholemeal wraps

a large handful of fresh watercress or lamb's lettuce

sea salt and freshly ground black pepper

SERVES 2

Heat half the coconut oil and all of the butter in a non-stick frying pan over a medium-high heat until melted. Add the red onion and shallot, season with a little salt and pepper, add the balsamic vinegar and cook for 5 minutes until slightly softened, stirring occasionally.

Reduce the heat to medium-low and cook for a further 30 minutes until completely softened and caramelised, stirring occasionally. Remove the steaks from the fridge to come up to room temperature.

When the onions are almost cooked, preheat a griddle pan over a high heat. Rub the steaks with the remaining coconut oil and season well with salt and pepper.

Cook on the hot griddle pan for around 2–3 minutes on each side for medium-rare, or longer depending on the thickness and how you like your steak cooked. Remove the steaks to a chopping board to rest for a few minutes.

Warm the wraps in the microwave for 30 seconds. Place a handful of fresh watercress or lamb's lettuce on each wrap, divide the caramelised onions between them, then slice the steak into small, thin strips and add to each wrap before folding.

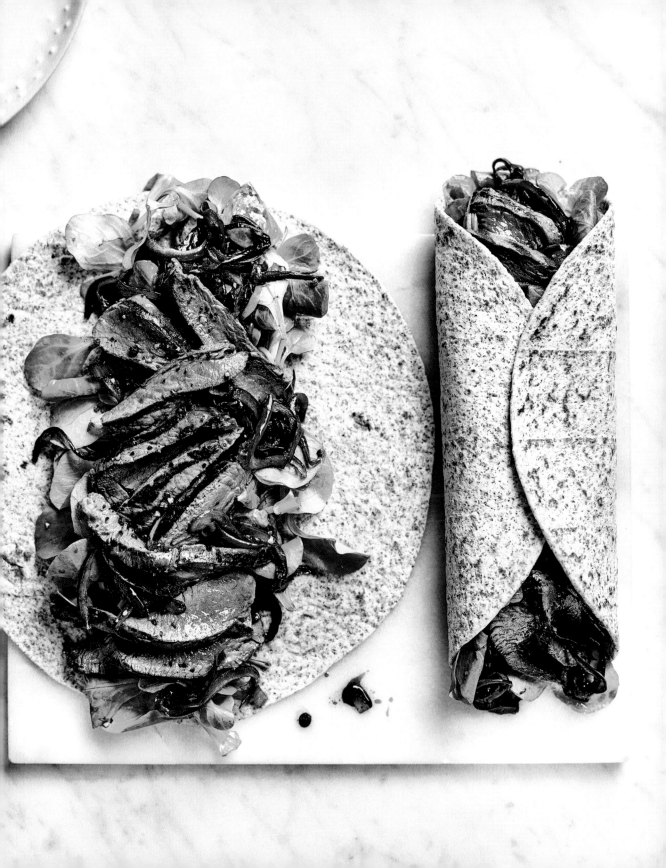

Warm Roasted Butternut Squash, Lentil and Feta Salad with Lemony Tahini Dressing

(GF) (V)

Providing perfect post-workout fuel, this delicious combination of protein, low GI carbohydrates and fats will ensure a slow release of energy so that you're not left starving at the 4pm slump.

1 tbsp coconut oil
200g butternut squash, peeled and cubed
250g Puy lentils
1 tbsp tahini
1 lemon, zested and juiced
1 small garlic clove, peeled and minced
50g feta, crumbled
a few fresh mint leaves
sea salt

SERVES 2

Preheat the oven to 180°C/350°F/Gas Mark 4.

Put the coconut oil into a roasting tray and place in the hot oven until melted. Remove and add the butternut squash with a pinch of sea salt, toss to coat and cook in the hot oven for around 35 minutes or until softened, tossing halfway through.

Meanwhile, cook the lentils according to the packet instructions, then drain.

Make the dressing by mixing the tahini with 2 tablespoons of water, the lemon juice, zest and garlic and stir until completely combined, adding extra water to loosen if needed.

Tip the lentils onto plates, and top with the roasted butternut squash chunks and feta.

Drizzle over the dressing, garnish with the mint leaves and serve.

Shredded Sprout, Bacon and Almond Salad

DF GF

Sprouts definitely aren't just for Christmas, and this super salad packed full of protein and vital nutrients such as vitamin C will help you stay in optimal health year round.

200g Brussels sprouts, trimmed
2 tbsp flaked almonds
1 tsp coconut oil
3 lean bacon medallions, thinly sliced
1 small lemon, zested and juiced
1 garlic clove, peeled and minced
1 tsp honey
1 tbsp extra virgin olive oil
sea salt and freshly ground black
    pepper

SERVES 1

Shred the Brussels sprouts in a food processor or thinly slice using a mandolin. Toast the almonds in a small dry frying pan over a medium heat until lightly golden, shaking the pan often, then tip onto a plate and leave to cool.

Heat the coconut oil in a large frying pan over a medium-high heat until melted, add the bacon and fry for a few minutes until crisp. Add the sprouts and lemon zest and cook for a further 3 minutes, or until the sprouts have softened.

Meanwhile, mix the lemon juice, garlic and honey with the olive oil and a pinch of salt and pepper until combined. Toss the sprouts and bacon in the lemony dressing and serve sprinkled with the toasted almonds.

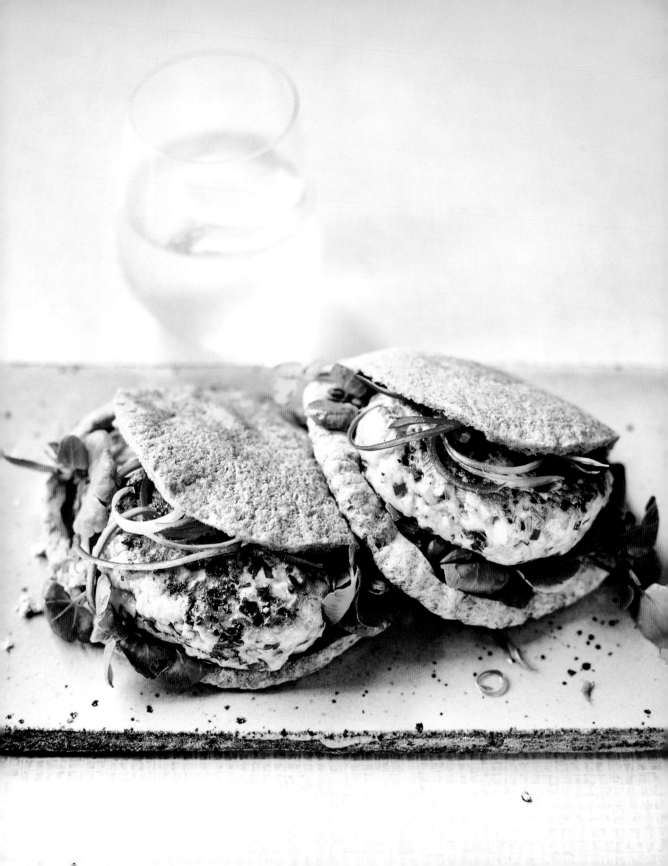

Thai-style Turkey Burgers

DF

These tasty burgers have a little chilli kick and are ideal to pop into a sealable container and take to work for lunch.

300g turkey mince

4 spring onions, 2 finely chopped, 2 sliced

1 red chilli, deseeded and finely chopped, plus extra slices

a small chunk of ginger, peeled and grated

1 free-range egg yolk

¼ of a bunch of fresh coriander, leaves chopped

1 tbsp coconut oil

2 wholemeal pitta breads

30g watercress

1 tomato, sliced (optional)

SERVES 2

In a bowl, mix the turkey mince, chopped spring onion, chopped chilli, ginger, egg yolk and most of the coriander until fully combined, then use your hands to form two burger patties.

Heat the coconut oil in a non-stick frying pan over a medium-high heat until melted. Fry the burgers for 5 minutes on each side until cooked through.

Toast the pitta breads and carefully slice open. Stuff with the watercress and place a burger in each. Finish with the sliced chilli, remaining coriander, sliced spring onion and sliced tomato, if using.

Souper Simple Broccoli Soup

(DF) (GF) (V)

Ideal for those chillier days, broccoli is an exceptionally rich source of vitamin C, so is ideal for helping to stave off any winter colds!

2 tbsp coconut oil

1 leek, trimmed and sliced

2 garlic cloves, peeled and minced

2 tsp ground cumin

1 vegetable stock cube

2 heads of broccoli, broken into small florets

a large handful of fresh spinach

400ml tinned coconut milk

sea salt and freshly ground black pepper

FOR THE TOPPING

3 tbsp pine nuts

1 garlic clove, peeled and minced

¼ tsp ground allspice

½ small lemon, juiced

2 tbsp tahini

1 tbsp extra virgin olive oil

SERVES 6

Heat the coconut oil in a large saucepan over a medium-low heat until melted. Add the sliced leek, cover with a lid and cook for around 10 minutes, until softened, stirring occasionally. Add the garlic and cumin, and cook for a further minute.

Dissolve the stock cube in 1.25 litres of boiling water. Pour into the pan, add the broccoli florets and bring to the boil. Turn the heat back down to medium-low and gently simmer for around 15 minutes. Add the spinach and coconut milk and simmer for a few minutes with the lid off until thickened and the spinach has wilted.

Meanwhile make the topping by toasting the pine nuts in a small dry frying pan over a medium heat until golden, shaking the pan often. Combine the minced garlic with the allspice, lemon juice, tahini, 2 tablespoons of water and a dash of extra virgin olive oil to make a creamy sauce.

Transfer the soup to a blender and blitz until smooth, or use a hand blender to purée, then season with salt and pepper to taste. Serve the soup topped with a tablespoon of the tahini sauce, loosened with water if needed, and sprinkle over the toasted pine nuts.

Mini Turkey Burger and Aubergine Bites

DF GF

A lighter twist on traditional sliders, these aubergine bites are the perfect simple swap and taste pretty darn good, too!

1½ tbsp coconut oil

2 large aubergines

250g lean turkey mince

1 red onion, peeled, halved and finely chopped

1 tsp paprika

1 tsp dried mixed herbs

1 free-range egg yolk

½ a bunch of fresh coriander, leaves chopped

2 large tomatoes

sea salt and freshly ground black pepper

SERVES 2

Preheat the oven to 200°C/400°F/Gas Mark 6. Line a large baking tray with greaseproof paper, put half the coconut oil on the tray and place in the oven until melted.

Slice each aubergine into 5mm rounds (you will need 12 slices altogether). Place on the lined baking tray and turn to coat in the coconut oil. Season lightly and cook in the hot oven for 35 minutes, turning halfway through.

In a bowl, mix the turkey mince, onion, paprika, mixed herbs, egg yolk and coriander with a pinch of sea salt and black pepper until completely combined. Use your hands, shape the mixture into six small burger patties, place on a plate and put into the fridge to firm up.

Slice each tomato into six and cook in the hot oven with the aubergine for the final 7 minutes. Heat the remainder of the coconut oil in a large non-stick frying pan over a medium-high heat until melted. Remove the patties from the fridge and fry for 5 minutes until cooked through, turning halfway through. You may need to do this in batches.

Layer up one slice of aubergine with one slice of tomato, place a turkey patty on top and sandwich with another slice of aubergine and tomato. I like to use cocktail sticks to hold the layers together.

Butternut Squash and Quinoa Chilli

GF **V**

This is one of my favourite combinations to prepare and take with me when I'm on the go. Full of slow-releasing carbohydrates, this dish will keep you feeling full of energy throughout your day.

70g quinoa, rinsed
1 tbsp coconut oil
1 red onion, peeled and finely diced
1 garlic clove, peeled and minced
1 tsp ground cumin
1 tsp chilli powder
400g butternut squash, peeled and cubed
800g tinned chopped tomatoes
200g tinned red kidney beans, drained
¼ of a bunch of fresh coriander, leaves chopped
1 red chilli, deseeded and finely sliced
Greek yoghurt, to serve

SERVES 2

Put the quinoa into a bowl, cover with boiling water and set aside to soak.

Heat the coconut oil in a large frying pan over a medium heat until melted. Add the onion and garlic and fry for 5–7 minutes until softened, stirring often and adding the spices for the final minute.

Add the butternut squash and cook for 5 minutes, then add the chopped tomatoes and simmer for 15 minutes.

Drain the quinoa and add to the pan along with a tin's worth of water. Bring to the boil, then simmer for a further 15 minutes, or until the squash is tender, adding a splash of water if needed.

Add the kidney beans for the final 2 minutes to warm through, then serve scattered with coriander, chilli and Greek yoghurt.

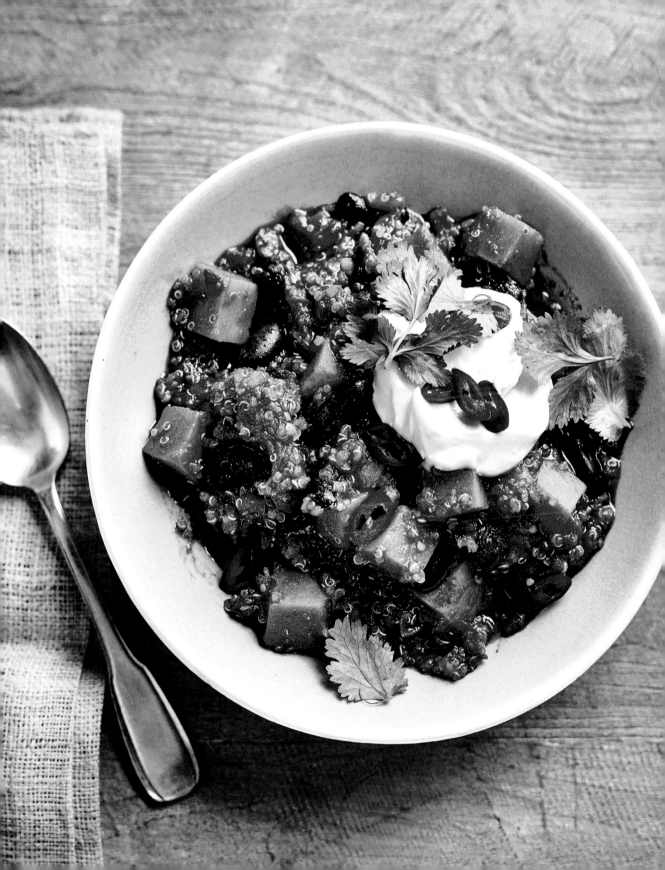

Super Seed Loaf

DF **GF** **V**

This loaf is my saviour. Perfect to freeze and defrost on those busy weeks.

coconut oil, for greasing
120g ground almonds
100g sunflower seeds
100g pumpkin seeds
75g sesame seeds
30g chia seeds
½ tsp sea salt
5 free-range eggs
75ml unsweetened almond milk

MAKES A 450G (1LB) LOAF

Preheat the oven to 180°C/350°F/Gas Mark 4. Grease and line a 450g (1lb) loaf tin.

Combine the ground almonds, sunflower seeds, pumpkin seeds, sesame seeds and chia seeds in a bowl with ½ a teaspoon of sea salt.

Crack the eggs into a separate bowl, whisk until fully combined, then add the almond milk. Slowly combine the wet with the dry ingredients, stirring continuously.

Pour the mixture into the lined tin and bake in the hot oven for 40 minutes, until risen, golden and firm to the touch. Transfer to a wire rack to cool.

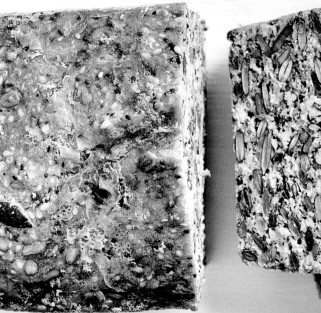
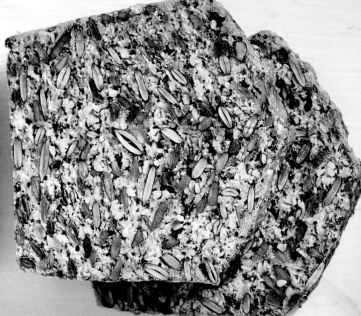

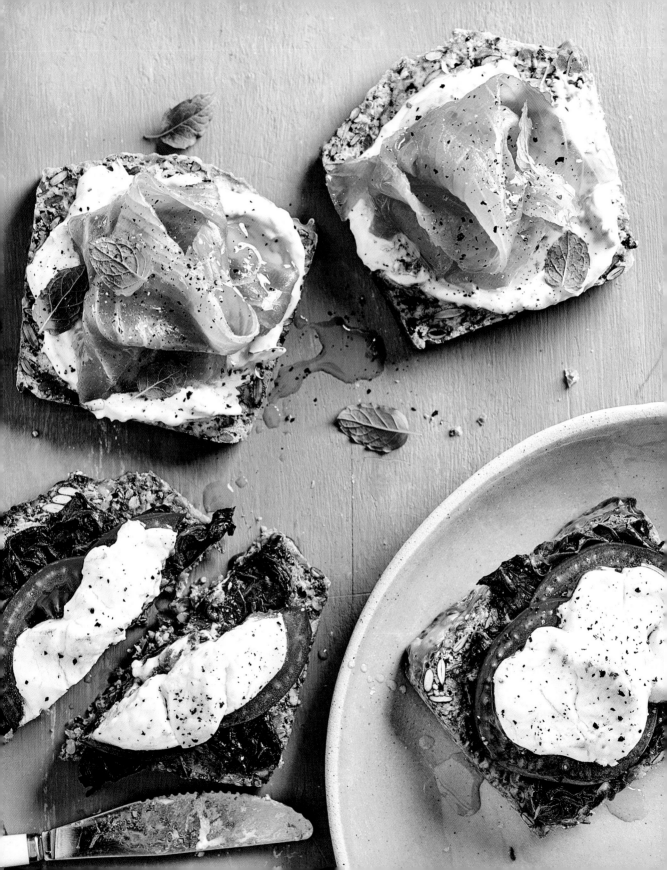

Super Seed Loaf with Goat's Cheese and Grilled Tomatoes

My Super Seed Loaf topped with deliciously creamy goat's cheese is an absolute winner.

½ tsp coconut oil
a handful of fresh spinach, chopped
2 slices of Super Seed Loaf (see recipe, page 102)
1 tomato, thinly sliced
40g goat's cheese, thinly sliced
freshly ground black pepper

SERVES 1

Heat the coconut oil in a frying pan over a medium heat until melted, add the spinach and cook until wilted, stirring often.

Preheat the grill to medium.

Top the slices of Super Seed Loaf with the wilted spinach, layer the sliced tomato and goat's cheese on top and season well with black pepper.

Place on a baking tray and cook under the hot grill for about 1–2 minutes, until the goat's cheese has melted.

Super Seed Loaf with Smoked Salmon and Minted Yoghurt

GF

Packed with healthy fats, this combination of delicious smoked salmon and minted yoghurt feels so indulgent, but is surprisingly simple, and you can knock it together in no time at all.

2 tbsp Greek yoghurt
½ lemon, juiced
a few fresh mint leaves, roughly chopped
½ tsp pesto (see recipe, page 109)
2 slices of Super Seed Loaf (see recipe, page 102)
80g smoked salmon
extra virgin olive oil, for drizzling
sea salt and freshly ground black pepper

SERVES 1

Mix the Greek yoghurt with the lemon juice and a good pinch of sea salt and black pepper. Add the chopped mint and pesto and mix well.

Top the slices of the Super Seed Loaf with the minted yogurt before tearing over the smoked salmon. Finish with another pinch of black pepper and a drizzle of olive oil.

Roasted Aubergine with Feta, Tahini, Pomegranate and Yoghurt

A simple combination of flavours and a source of dietary fibre. Aubergine is an awesome ingredient to include in your diet.

2 medium aubergines
4 tbsp Greek yoghurt
60g feta, crumbled
a few sprigs of fresh coriander, leaves chopped
½ lemon, juiced
a few sprigs of fresh mint, chopped
2 tbsp coconut oil
1 tsp sumac
1 tbsp tahini
75g pomegranate seeds
sea salt and freshly ground black pepper

SERVES 2

Preheat the oven to 200°C/400°F/Gas Mark 6.

Halve the aubergines, use a knife to make criss-cross incisions into the flesh, season lightly with sea salt and set aside for at least 10 minutes.

Meanwhile, combine the Greek yoghurt with the crumbled feta, coriander and lemon juice in a bowl. Stir in most of the mint, season lightly with salt and black pepper and place in the fridge.

Heat the coconut oil in a small saucepan over a medium heat until melted. Remove from the heat and mix in the sumac.

Once slightly cooled, pour the sumac mixture over the aubergine and use your hands to rub the mixture over the aubergine halves, to coat. Season well, and roast in the hot oven for around 40 minutes, or until soft.

Meanwhile, mix the tahini with 2 tablespoons of water, adding more water if needed to create a drizzling consistency.

Serve the aubergine topped with the yoghurt and feta mixture, sprinkle over the pomegranate seeds, drizzle with the tahini and sprinkle with the remaining mint.

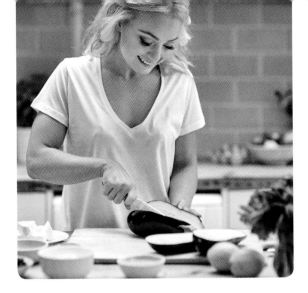
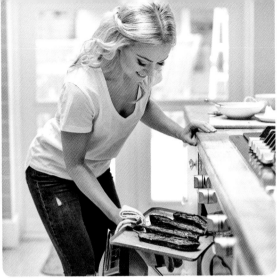
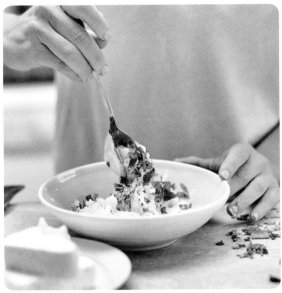
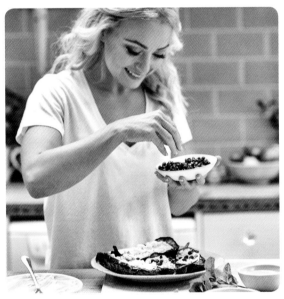
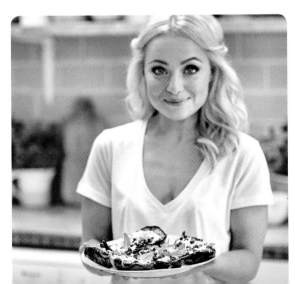
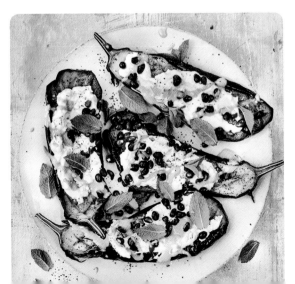

Gooey Goat's Cheese Scramble in Portobello Mushrooms

GF V

I couldn't resist sneaking in one of my all-time favourite combinations. A low-carb simple swap, these stuffed mushrooms are an any-time-of-the-day delicious dish.

4 large portobello mushrooms
2 tbsp coconut oil
4 free-range eggs
60g goat's cheese
¼ of a bunch of fresh chives, chopped
1 tsp butter
sea salt and freshly ground black
    pepper

SERVES 2

Preheat the oven to 200°C/400°F/Gas Mark 6. Line a baking tray with greaseproof paper.

Remove the stalks from the mushrooms and discard. Place the mushrooms on the lined baking tray.

Put the coconut oil into a small bowl and heat in the microwave until melted. Drizzle over the mushrooms and roast in the hot oven for 15–20 minutes, until cooked through.

About 5 minutes before the mushrooms are cooked, crack the eggs into a bowl and whisk until fully combined. Chop the goat's cheese into small chunks, add to the bowl with the chopped chives then season well with salt and pepper.

Melt the butter in a non-stick frying pan over a medium-low heat. Add the eggs to the pan and use a wooden spoon to scramble until cooked to your liking.

Serve the goat's cheese scramble in the upturned mushrooms.

Homemade Pesto Courgetti with Baked Cod

GF

A deliciously simple low-carb lunch that's packed full of flavour. The addition of pine nuts is my favourite part, providing a rich dose of monounsaturated fats.

1 tsp coconut oil
2 skinless, boneless cod fillets
10 cherry tomatoes, halved
2 large courgettes
sea salt and freshly ground black
    pepper

FOR THE PESTO
15g pine nuts
25g fresh basil
15g Parmesan cheese, plus extra
    to serve
1 small garlic clove, peeled and minced
50ml extra virgin olive oil

SERVES 2

Preheat the oven to 200°C/400°F/Gas Mark 6 and line a baking tray with foil. Put the coconut oil into a small bowl and heat in the microwave until melted.

Lay the cod and tomatoes on the lined tray and drizzle over the coconut oil, tossing the tomatoes gently to coat. Season well with a good pinch of salt and pepper and cook in the hot oven for around 10–12 minutes, until the fish is just cooked.

To make the pesto, toast the pine nuts in a small frying pan over a medium heat until golden, shaking the pan often, then set aside to cool.

Put the cooled pine nuts into a food processor with the basil, Parmesan, garlic and olive oil and blitz to your desired pesto consistency.

Use a spiralizer or julienne peeler to create courgetti or use a vegetable peeler to peel the courgettes into long ribbons, avoiding the seeds. Place the courgetti and pesto in a bowl and mix until completely combined.

When the cod is cooked, divide the courgetti between two plates – you can steam the courgetti for a couple of minutes first, if you prefer. Top with the cooked tomatoes and cod and finish with shavings of Parmesan.

Mushroom and Mozzarella Shakshuka

GF V

This is a delicious alternative to the classic shakshuka. Featuring the always delicious gooey mozzarella, it's an absolute winner of a dish!

2 tbsp coconut oil

1 large red onion, peeled, halved and diced

1 garlic clove, peeled and minced

15 button mushrooms, halved

1 tsp smoked paprika

½ tsp ground cumin

½ aubergine, chopped

400g tinned chopped tomatoes

4 free-range eggs

100g mozzarella, cut into chunks

¼ of a bunch of fresh coriander, leaves chopped

sea salt and freshly ground black pepper

SERVES 2

Begin by heating the coconut oil in a large non-stick frying pan over a medium-low heat until melted.

Add the onion, garlic, mushrooms, spices, aubergine and a pinch of salt and pepper and cook for 15 minutes, stirring occasionally.

Add the chopped tomatoes and cook for a further 15 minutes, stirring occasionally.

Using a spoon, make four shallow wells in the tomato sauce, then crack an egg into each well.

Evenly scatter over the mozzarella, cover with a lid and continue to cook until the egg whites have set and the egg yolks are cooked to your liking.

Serve scattered with the chopped coriander.

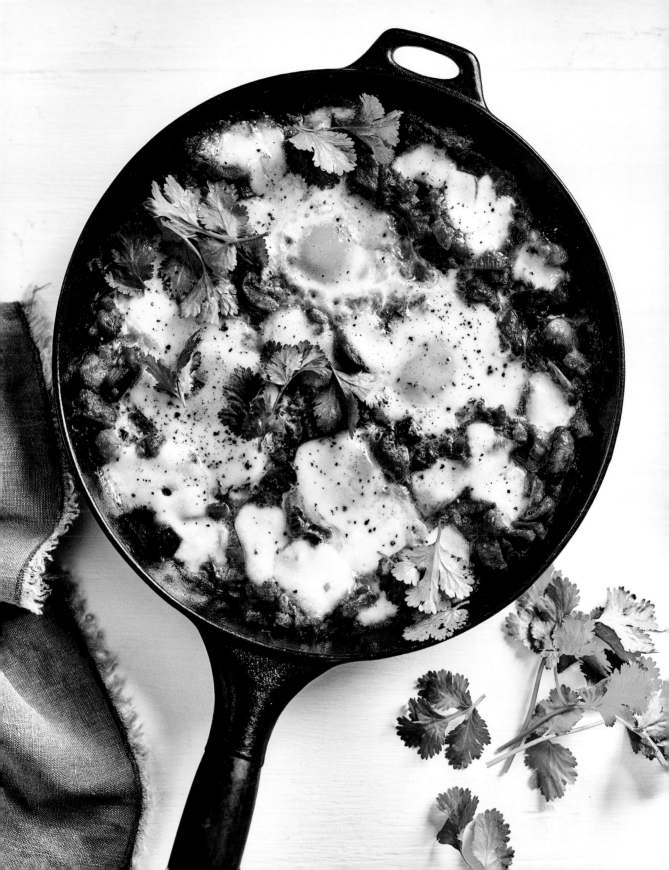

Salmon and Mango Ceviche

GF **DF**

Perfect for warm summer days.

250g skinless sushi-grade salmon fillet
1 ripe mango, peeled, halved and
  stoned
1½ limes, zested and juiced
1½ tbsp extra virgin olive oil
1½ red chillies, deseeded and finely
  sliced
sea salt and freshly ground black
  pepper

SERVES 2

Lightly sprinkle the salmon with sea salt and set aside for around 10 minutes. Thinly slice the mango.

Rinse the salt from the salmon, pat dry with kitchen paper, then thinly slice and place in a bowl. In another bowl, mix together the lime juice, olive oil, and most of the lime zest and chilli with a pinch of salt and pepper. Pour two-thirds of the marinade over the salmon and stir to coat.

Divide the coated salmon and mango evenly between two plates so that the slices are overlapping. Drizzle with the remaining marinade, sprinkle over the remaining lime zest and chilli and eat immediately.

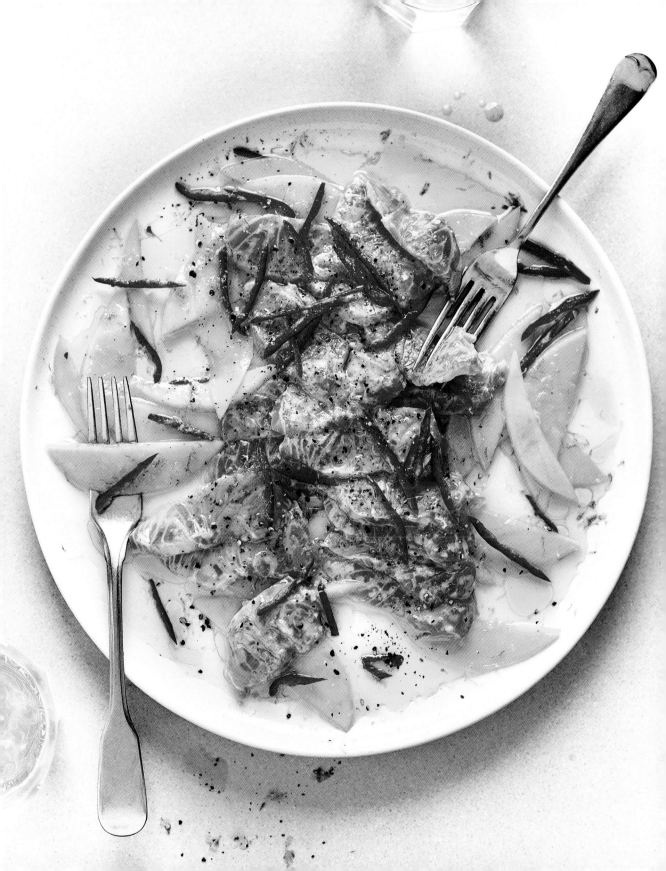

Sweet Potato and Tenderstem Broccoli Frittata

(GF) (V)

With sweet potatoes providing an awesome dose of vitamin A, this nutrient-packed dish not only tastes great, but is a brilliant way of incorporating this delicious veg into your diet.

1 small sweet potato (about 250g),
    peeled and chopped
100g Tenderstem broccoli
1 tbsp coconut oil
1 garlic clove, peeled and minced
4 free-range eggs
40g feta, crumbled
sea salt and freshly ground black
    pepper

SERVES 2

Put the sweet potato into a medium saucepan, cover with cold water and bring to the boil over a high heat. Reduce the heat to low and simmer for 15–20 minutes, adding the broccoli for the final 5 minutes. Drain and leave to steam dry.

Preheat the grill to medium.

Heat the coconut oil in a large frying pan over a medium heat until melted. Add the minced garlic along with the sweet potato and broccoli and cook for 1 minute, stirring regularly.

Meanwhile, crack the eggs into a bowl, whisk until fully combined, then season well with salt and pepper.

Ensure the veg in the pan is evenly spread out, then pour in the whisked eggs. Once the bottom has set, spread the feta evenly across the top and place the pan under the grill for 2–5 minutes until set and cooked through.

Shredded Veggie Slaw with Avocado and Sunflower Seeds

Combining a rainbow of veggies and healthy fats, this super salad has an amazing nutrient profile that will nourish you from the inside out.

2 large carrots, peeled
½ red cabbage
1 small apple, halved and cored
1 large beetroot, peeled, trimmed and
    halved
30g sunflower seeds
75ml extra virgin olive oil
35ml apple cider vinegar
1 tsp honey
1 avocado, peeled, stoned and chopped
sea salt and freshly ground black
    pepper

SERVES 2

Grate the carrots, red cabbage, apple and beetroot on a box grater or using the grater attachment on a food processor, then tip into a mixing bowl.

Lightly toast the sunflower seeds in a small dry frying pan over a medium heat for a couple of minutes until lightly golden, shaking the pan often. Remove from the heat and set aside to cool.

Next, prepare the dressing by mixing the olive oil with the cider vinegar, honey, 1 tablespoon of water and season with salt and pepper.

Pour two-thirds of the dressing over the shredded veggies and toss to coat. Divide between two plates, scatter over the avocado and toasted sunflower seeds, then pour over the remaining dressing and serve.

Wild Rice, Roasted Chickpea and Harissa Chicken Salad

DF GF

This, for me, is a perfect prep-ahead meal, and makes for an awesome cook once, eat twice dish that you can pop into a container and take on the go. It tastes pretty good, too!

2 tbsp coconut oil
1 tsp ground cumin
1 tsp smoked paprika
½ tsp chilli powder
400g tinned chickpeas, drained
150g wild rice, rinsed
1 tsp harissa paste
2 skinless, boneless chicken breasts,
    cut into strips
2 large handfuls of rocket
2 tbsp pomegranate seeds
¼ of a bunch of fresh coriander, leaves
    chopped
sea salt and freshly ground black
    pepper

FOR THE DRESSING
1 garlic clove, peeled and minced
½ lemon, juiced
2 tbsp extra virgin olive oil
sea salt and freshly ground black
    pepper

SERVES 2

Preheat the oven to 200°C/400°F/Gas Mark 6. Line a baking tray with greaseproof paper. Put 1 tablespoon of coconut oil into a large bowl and heat in the microwave until melted.

Stir the spices into the melted coconut oil, add the chickpeas and stir to fully coat. Tip onto the lined baking tray and season with salt and pepper. Spread out evenly and roast in the hot oven for around 30–35 minutes, until crisp.

Meanwhile, make the dressing by combining the garlic, lemon juice and olive oil and season well with salt and pepper.

Cook the rice according to the packet instructions and place in a bowl.

Put the remaining tablespoon of coconut oil into the bowl used for the chickpeas and heat in the microwave until melted, then leave to cool slightly. Mix the harissa into the cooled melted coconut oil, then add the chicken and use your hands to coat the chicken in the mix.

Place a large frying pan over a medium-high heat. Transfer the chicken into the pan and fry for about 5–7 minutes, until completely cooked through, stirring occasionally.

When the chickpeas are cooked, mix with the wild rice so that the spicy flavours from the chickpeas combine.

Divide the rocket between two plates, top with the rice and chickpea mixure, then top with the cooked chicken. Scatter over the pomegranate seeds and coriander, pour over the dressing and serve.

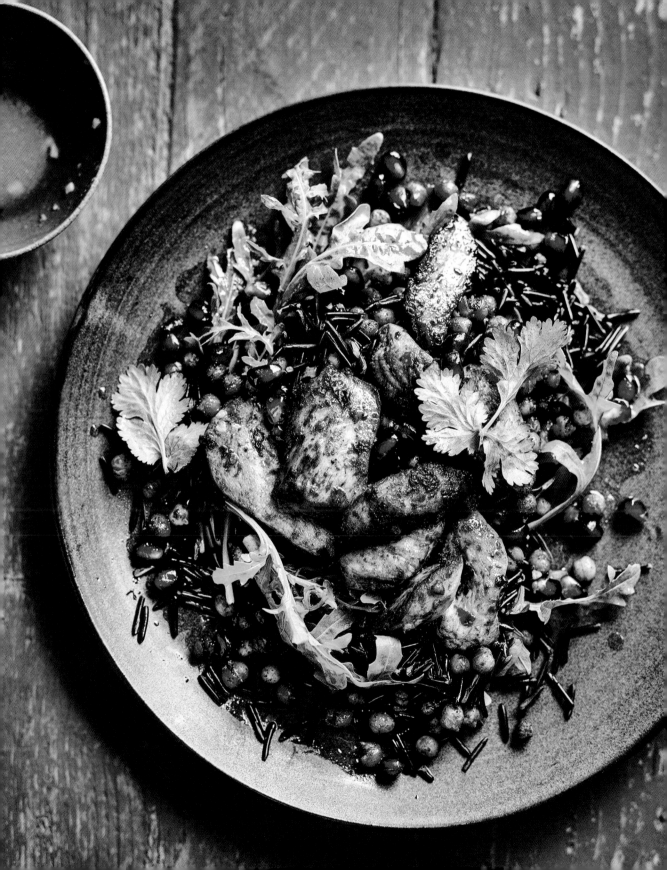

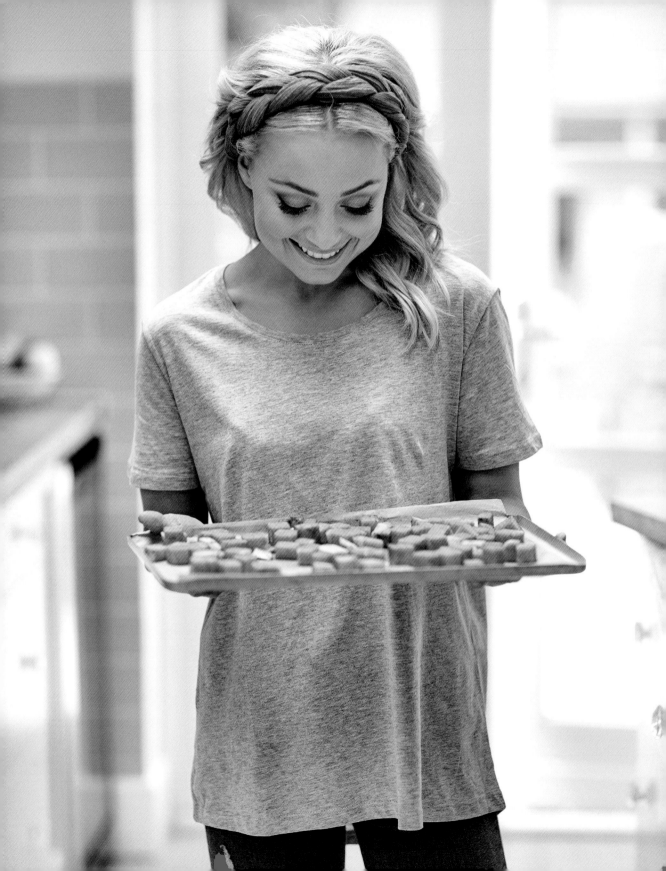

DINNER

Venison Steak with Soy, Pomegranate and Ginger and Miso-glazed Parsnip Fries

DF

Venison is particularly rich in iron. Paired with these sweet roasties, this nutrient-dense dish is perfect for repairing muscles post workout.

1 tbsp extra virgin olive oil

a chunk of ginger, peeled and grated

1 garlic clove, peeled and minced

2 tbsp soy sauce

1 tbsp pomegranate molasses

2 venison steaks (around 200g each)

2 tbsp coconut oil

300g parsnips, peeled and cut into 5cm batons

1 tbsp miso paste

2 handfuls of fresh baby spinach, chopped

sea salt and freshly ground black pepper

SERVES 2

Preheat the oven to 200°C/400°F/Gas Mark 6.

In a bowl, mix together the olive oil, ginger, garlic, soy sauce and pomegranate molasses. Add the venison steaks, turn to coat and set aside to marinate for about 15 minutes.

Put half the coconut oil into a roasting tray and place in the oven to melt. Once melted, remove the tray from the oven, tip in the parsnips along with the miso paste and toss to coat.

Season with pepper (it doesn't need much salt, as miso is already quite salty – you can always add some once cooked if needed) and cook in the hot oven for about 40 minutes, tossing halfway through.

Meanwhile, heat the remaining tablespoon of coconut oil in a frying pan over a medium-high heat until melted. Add the venison steaks and cook for around 3–4 minutes on each side for medium-rare, or longer depending on their thickness and how you like them cooked. Remove the steaks to a chopping board to rest for a few minutes. Return the pan to a high heat. Pour in the leftover marinade and leave it to bubble until thickened.

Slice and serve the steak alongside the parsnips and chopped spinach, then drizzle with the reduced marinade.

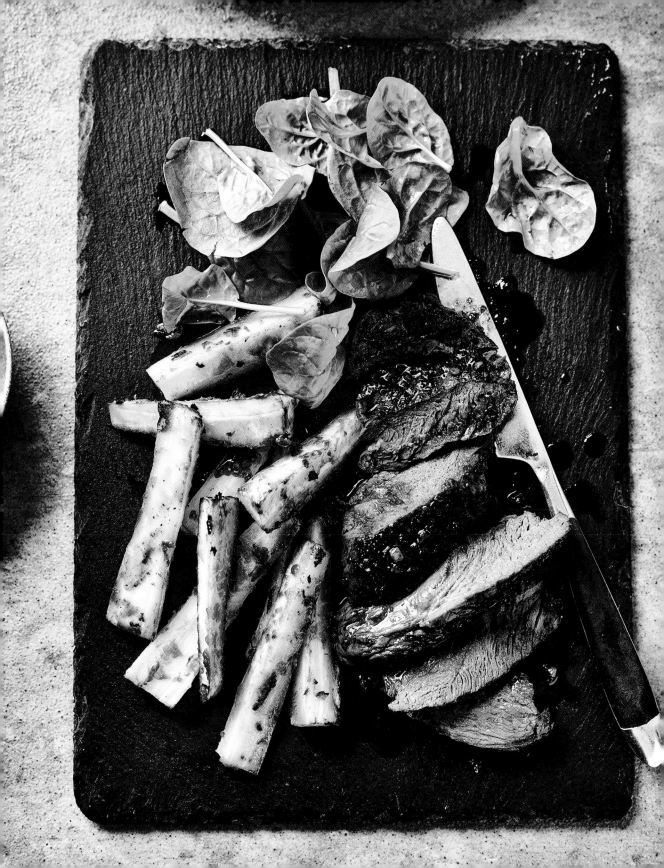

Griddled Prawn Skewers with a Harissa and Honey Dressing

DF GF

Sweet and spicy, these remind me of a takeaway without the added nasties! The perfect light dinner to finish the day.

2 tsp harissa paste
2 tsp honey
½ lemon, juiced
150g raw king prawns
1 tbsp coconut oil
1 red pepper, halved, deseeded and sliced
½ red onion, peeled, halved and finely chopped
8 baby plum tomatoes, halved
150g pre-cooked quinoa
¼ of a bunch of fresh coriander, leaves chopped
sea salt and freshly ground black pepper

SERVES 2

In a bowl, mix the harissa, honey and lemon juice. In another bowl, toss the prawns in half the harissa mixture to fully coat.

Heat half the coconut oil in a frying pan over a medium-high heat until melted. Add the pepper and red onion and fry for 7–10 minutes, until softened, adding the tomatoes halfway through and stirring often. Heat the quinoa according to the packet instructions, tip into a bowl and stir through the peppers, tomatoes and red onion.

Heat the remaining ½ tablespoon of coconut oil on a griddle pan over a medium-high heat until melted.

Thread the prawns evenly onto skewers (if you are using wooden skewers, soak them in water for 20 minutes before using), then place on the griddle pan to cook for about 3–4 minutes, turning every minute, until cooked through.

Stir the coriander through the quinoa and season generously.

Serve the prawns with the quinoa and drizzle with the remaining harissa and honey dressing.

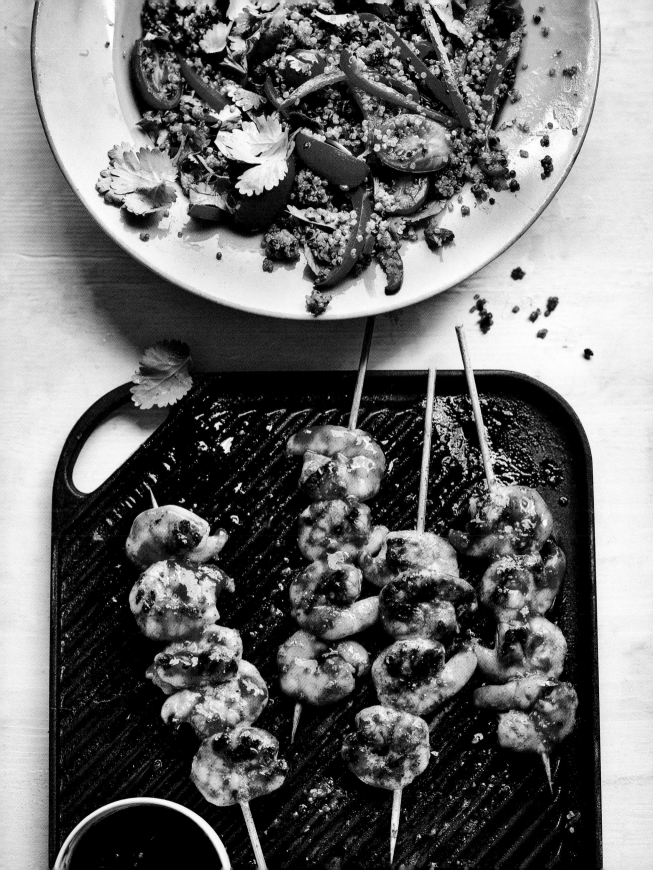

Maple Syrup and Pistachio-crusted Salmon with Tenderstem Broccoli

DF GF

A surprise flavour combination that provides an excellent source of omega-3s, this dish feels like sophisticated dining without the fuss.

coconut oil, for greasing
20g pistachio nuts, shelled
1 tbsp maple syrup
½ lime, juiced
½ tsp Dijon mustard
2 salmon fillets
200g Tenderstem broccoli
sea salt and freshly ground black
    pepper

SERVES 2

Preheat the oven to 200°C/400°F/Gas Mark 6. Line a baking tray with foil and lightly grease with coconut oil.

Chop the pistachio nuts. In a mixing bowl, combine the maple syrup, lime juice and Dijon mustard, and season with a pinch of salt and pepper. Add the salmon fillets and turn to coat.

Place the salmon fillets on the lined tray, top with the chopped pistachio nuts and pour over any remaining maple syrup mixture. Cook in the hot oven for about 12–15 minutes, until the salmon is just cooked.

Meanwhile, steam the broccoli for 5–7 minutes until tender, then serve with the salmon.

Chilli and Lime Chicken with Grilled Tomatoes and Guacamole

GF

Avocados are an excellent source of vitamin E, which helps to protect our bodies against damage.

1 lime, juiced and zested

1 garlic clove, peeled and crushed

¼ of a bunch of fresh coriander, leaves chopped

1 red chilli, halved and deseeded

1 tbsp extra virgin olive oil, plus extra for greasing

2 skinless, boneless chicken breasts

a pinch of dried chilli flakes

1 avocado, peeled, halved and stoned

1 tbsp Greek yoghurt

2 large tomatoes, sliced

sea salt and freshly ground black pepper

SERVES 2

First, make the marinade. In a small blender, blitz half the lime juice, all the lime zest, half the garlic, half the coriander and all the fresh chilli with the extra virgin olive oil. If you don't have a small blender you can do this step by hand, by grinding the ingredients in a pestle and mortar.

Pour the marinade into a bowl, add the chicken breasts, turn to coat and set aside to marinate for about 30 minutes.

Now make the guacamole. In a large bowl, mix together the remaining garlic, lime juice, coriander and the chilli flakes. Add the avocado flesh with the yoghurt and use a fork to mash until fully combined. Season with a little salt and pepper.

Preheat the grill to medium. Line two baking trays with foil and lightly oil. Lay the tomatoes on one of the lined trays and season with salt and pepper. Cook under the hot grill for around 3–5 minutes, turning halfway through.

Place the marinated chicken breasts on the other lined tray and cook under the hot grill for 10 minutes, or until cooked through, turning halfway through.

Serve the chicken with the grilled tomatoes and a big tablespoon of guacamole.

Creamy Puy Lentils with Peas, Feta and Bacon

GF

Lentils provide an excellent source of protein, and are a low-GI source of carbohydrates that I include in my diet a lot. This warm salad makes for the perfect dinner; you can pop it in a sealable container for the next day, too.

1 tbsp coconut oil

4 lean bacon medallions, roughly chopped

1 red onion, peeled, halved and finely diced

200g Puy lentils, rinsed

50g frozen peas

1 tbsp balsamic vinegar

200g cherry tomatoes, halved

100g Greek yoghurt

50g feta, crumbled

a few fresh mint leaves, finely chopped

sea salt and freshly ground black pepper

SERVES 2

Heat ½ a tablespoon of coconut oil in a frying pan over a medium-high heat until melted and fry the bacon for 5–7 minutes or until crisp and cooked through, turning halfway through. Remove from the pan, and pat with kitchen paper to remove any excess fat.

Return the pan to the heat, add the remaining coconut oil and fry the red onion for around 5–7 minutes, until softened, stirring occasionally.

Next, add half the bacon, all the lentils and pour in enough boiling water to cover the lentils completely. Bring to the boil, cover, reduce the heat to medium-low and simmer for 20 minutes.

Remove the lid, add the peas, remaining bacon, balsamic vinegar and tomatoes and season well with salt and pepper. By this point the majority of the water should have been absorbed. Cook for a further 5 minutes over a medium heat.

Finally, remove from the heat and set aside to cool for a few minutes. Stir through the Greek yoghurt and top with the crumbled feta and fresh mint.

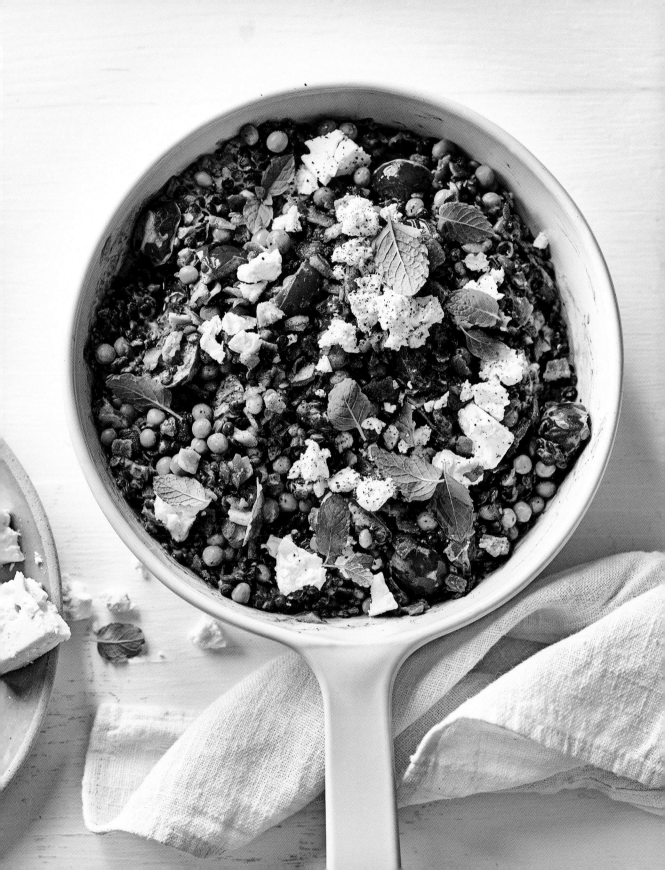

Kale Pesto-baked Cod

DF GF

I love creating pesto variations and my kale pesto is one of my favourites. With kale being one of the most nutrient-dense foods around, this pesto is an excellent simple swap.

2 handfuls of kale, any large stems removed
40g almonds
40g cashew nuts
30g pine nuts
3 tbsp extra virgin olive oil, plus extra for greasing
2 tbsp apple cider vinegar
1 lemon, juiced
a few sprigs of basil, leaves chopped
2 skinless, boneless cod fillets
sea salt and freshly ground black pepper

SERVES 2

Steam the kale for 2 minutes until slightly wilted. Place the almonds, cashew nuts and pine nuts in a food processor and blitz for around 10 seconds.

Add the steamed kale, olive oil, cider vinegar, half the lemon juice, all the basil and a pinch of salt and pepper and further blitz to your desired pesto consistency, adding 50ml water to loosen if needed.

Preheat the oven to 180°C/350°F/Gas Mark 4. Line a baking tray with foil and lightly oil.

Place the cod on the lined tray and top the fillets with a generous helping of the pesto and an extra squeeze of lemon juice. Bake in the oven for around 10–12 minutes, until the fish is just cooked. Serve with your favourite veggie side.

Green and Lean Super Salad with Creamy Cashew Dressing

GF V

I absolutely love this dish on warm summer evenings when I don't fancy cooking in a hot kitchen! Packed full of micronutrients and antioxidant-rich blueberries, this salad will definitely help you feel good both inside and out.

50g cashew nuts

100g fresh spinach, chopped

100g kale, any large stems removed, chopped

1 tbsp extra virgin olive oil

½ red onion, peeled, halved and finely diced

1 red chilli, halved, deseeded and finely sliced

1 red pepper, halved, deseeded and cut into chunks

8–10 baby plum tomatoes, halved

1 lime, juiced

30g pumpkin seeds

1 avocado, peeled, halved and stoned

100g blueberries

50g feta, cut into chunks

sea salt and freshly ground black pepper

SERVES 2

The night before, tip the cashew nuts into a small bowl, cover with cold water and set aside to soak.

Begin prepping your salad by tossing the chopped spinach and kale in ½ tablespoon of the olive oil in a large salad bowl until completely coated.

Add the red onion, chilli, red pepper and tomatoes along with half the lime juice and the remaining ½ tablespoon of olive oil. Season well with salt and pepper and toss everything together.

Place the pumpkin seeds in a small frying pan over a medium-high heat and toast until golden and lightly popping, shaking the pan often. Remove from the heat and set aside.

Chop the avocado and scatter over the salad along with the blueberries, feta and toasted pumpkin seeds.

Finally, drain the cashew nuts and place them in a food processor or blender with the remaining lime juice, one or two splashes of water and some seasoning. Blitz until smooth, then pour over the finished salad.

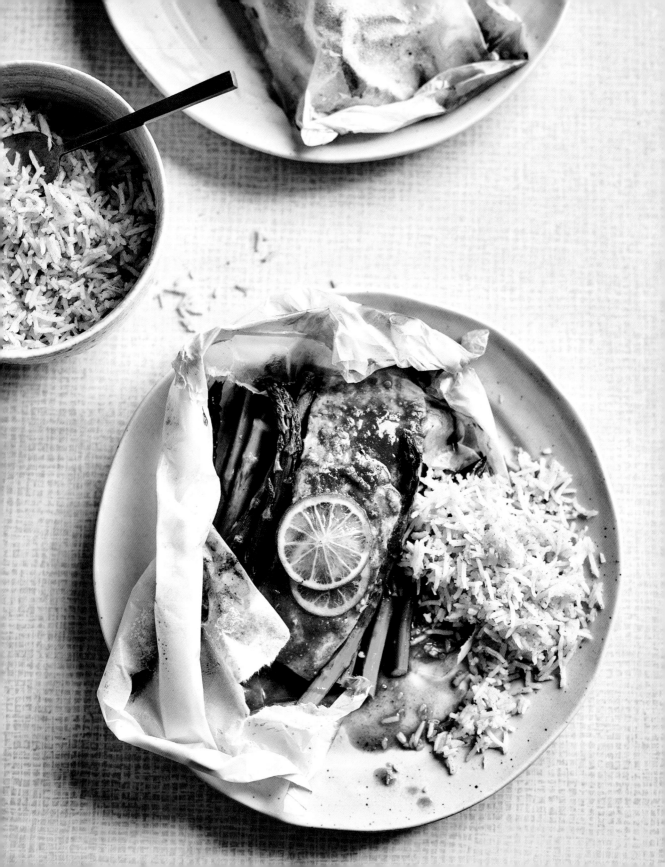

Harissa and Lime Salmon Parcels with Coconut Rice

DF GF

Simple, spicy and succulent salmon with deliciously sweet coconut rice is the perfect combination.

2 salmon fillets
200g asparagus
1 tsp coconut oil
1 tbsp harissa paste
1½ limes, ½ juiced and zested,
    ½ sliced, ½ cut into wedges
1 tbsp extra virgin olive oil
250g rice
20g desiccated coconut
¼ tsp paprika
sea salt and freshly ground black
    pepper

SERVES 2

Preheat the oven to 200°C/400°F/Gas Mark 6.

Tear off two large pieces of foil or greaseproof paper. Place a salmon fillet in the centre of each piece.

Snap the ends off the asparagus and, using your hands, rub the asparagus with the coconut oil until completely covered. Season with salt and pepper and arrange around each salmon fillet.

In a bowl, mix the harissa, lime juice, olive oil and a little salt and pepper and pour over the salmon. Top with the lime zest and two slices of lime.

Wrap the salmon tightly in the foil or greaseproof paper, sealing well. Place on a baking tray and cook in the hot oven for 18–20 minutes.

Meanwhile, cook the rice according to the packet instructions. Once cooked, stir through the desiccated coconut and paprika and season with salt and pepper. Serve the salmon parcels with the rice and a wedge of lime for squeezing over.

Loaded Sweet Potato Skins, Two Ways

You really can't beat stuffed sweet potatoes and this nutrient-dense vegetable is so versatile.

2 sweet potatoes (about 300–350g each)

SERVES 2

Preheat the oven to 200°C/400°F/Gas Mark 6. Line a baking sheet with greaseproof paper.

Carefully make small insertions in the sweet potatoes using a knife or fork. Place on the lined baking sheet and cook in the hot oven for 45 minutes–1 hour, or until completely soft.

While the potatoes are cooking, make your filling:

Smoked Mackerel, Yoghurt and Dill

Mackerel is one of my go-to foods for a dose of omega-3s – something I try to get into my diet every day – and this dish is the most delicious way to enjoy this oily fish.

2 small mackerel fillets, skin removed
4 tbsp Greek yoghurt
1 tsp wholegrain mustard
1 tbsp fresh dill, finely chopped
a pinch of paprika
1 lemon, ½ juiced, ½ cut into wedges
2 large handfuls of watercress
sea salt and freshly ground black pepper

Flake the mackerel into a bowl, add the Greek yoghurt, mustard, dill, paprika and lemon juice, season well with salt and pepper and use a fork to mix well.

When the sweet potatoes are cooked, carefully slice into the centre and stuff with the mackerel mixture. Serve with a handful of fresh watercress and lemon wedges for squeezing over, if you like.

Roasted Fig, Honey and Goat's Cheese

GF **V**

Another sweet and light variation, this gooey, indulgent dish includes figs, which are one of my favourite fruits. They are also rich in soluble fibre and are a great source of potassium.

1 tsp coconut oil
2 small fresh figs, quartered
100g goat's cheese
a pinch of ground cinnamon
a pinch of ground nutmeg
2 tsp honey, plus extra for drizzling
sea salt and freshly ground black
    pepper

Put the coconut oil into a small bowl and heat in the microwave until melted. Line a baking tray with foil.

About 10 minutes before the potatoes are cooked, place the figs on the lined tray, drizzle with the melted coconut oil, season with a pinch of sea salt and black pepper and cook in the hot oven for the final 10 minutes.

Carefully scoop out the inside of the potatoes using a spoon, aiming to keep the skin intact, and place in a bowl. Chop the goat's cheese and add most to the potato with a pinch of cinnamon and nutmeg, the honey and a little salt and pepper. Stir to combine and stuff the mixture carefully back into the potato skins.

Preheat the grill to medium. Top the sweet potatoes with the remaining goat's cheese and pop under the hot grill until melted. Top with the cooked figs and an extra drizzle of honey, if you like.

Everyday Chicken with Roasted Butternut Squash, Lime and Chilli

(GF)

A simple everyday dish that is full of flavour. This is perfect for cooking once and eating twice, so that's dinner and tomorrow's lunch sorted!

FOR THE CHICKEN

½ tsp paprika
½ tsp dried Italian seasoning
¼ tsp sea salt
¼ tsp freshly ground black pepper
¼ tsp garlic powder
a pinch of cayenne pepper
1 tbsp olive oil
2 large skinless, boneless chicken breasts

FOR THE SQUASH

300g butternut squash, peeled and diced
1 tbsp olive oil
1 tsp ground allspice
10g tahini
50g Greek yoghurt
½ lime, juiced
100g fresh spinach, chopped
1 red chilli, deseeded and thinly sliced

SERVES 2

Preheat the oven to 200°C/400°F/Gas Mark 6.

Begin with the chicken; in a bowl, mix the paprika, dried Italian seasoning, salt and pepper, garlic powder and cayenne pepper with the olive oil and stir until completely combined.

Add the chicken, turn to coat and place in the fridge to marinate for 30 minutes.

Meanwhile, for the squash, line a baking tray with greaseproof paper.

Tip the squash onto the tray. Pour over the olive oil, sprinkle over the allspice and toss to coat. Cook in the hot oven for 10 minutes.

Tear off two large pieces of foil and wrap each individual chicken breast tightly in the foil. After the squash has been cooking for 10 minutes, place the wrapped chicken parcels beside them and cook for a further 25 minutes, or until the squash is tender and the chicken is cooked through.

While the chicken and squash are cooking, mix together the tahini, Greek yoghurt, lime juice, a pinch of sea salt and 1 teaspoon of water and set aside.

Divide the spinach between two plates. Top each with a chicken breast, half the butternut squash and a dollop of the tahini and lime sauce, finally finishing with a sprinkling of fresh chilli.

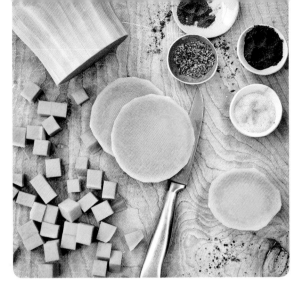
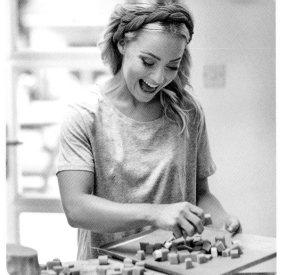
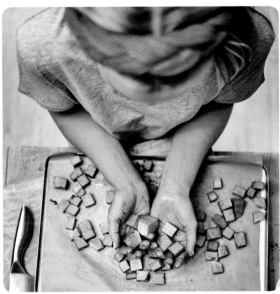
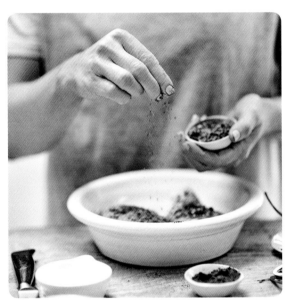
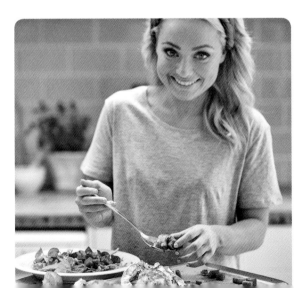
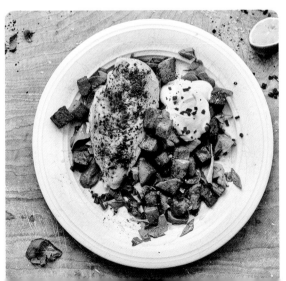

Griddled Steak with Balsamic Puy Lentils and Feta

Steak is serious soul food. It is full of protein and iron, a mineral many of us can become deficient in, and this combination is a delicious way of ensuring that you're getting a good dose of this vital nutrient.

2 quality, thick rump or sirloin steaks

1 tbsp olive oil

1 garlic clove, peeled and finely chopped

1 red chilli, deseeded and finely sliced

1 tbsp balsamic vinegar

250g packet of pre-cooked Puy lentils

a small handful of fresh mint, finely chopped

100g fresh spinach, roughly chopped

50g feta, sliced into chunks

sea salt and freshly ground black pepper

SERVES 2

30 minutes before you're ready to cook, remove the steaks from the fridge to come up to room temperature.

Rub the steaks on either side with half the olive oil and season well with salt and pepper. Heat a griddle pan over a high heat until very hot.

Cook the steaks on the hot griddle pan for around 2–3 minutes on each side for medium-rare, or longer depending on their thickness and how you like them cooked. Remove the steaks to a chopping board to rest for a few minutes.

Return the pan to a medium-low heat. Add the remaining olive oil along with the garlic and half the chilli. Cook for about a minute, add the balsamic vinegar, stir well and then pour into a bowl.

Heat the lentils according to the packet instructions and tip into a bowl. Add the chopped mint, pour over the balsamic dressing, add any juices from the rested steak and season with salt and pepper if needed. Finally, add the chopped spinach, toss everything together and add the feta chunks.

Slice the steaks into thin strips, serve with the lentil salad and top with the remaining chilli.

Citrus Baked Salmon with Broccoli Pesto

GF **DF**

Another of my favourite pesto variations, broccoli is a great source of fibre, which helps contribute towards regulating digestive health.

2 salmon fillets
1 lemon, ½ juiced, ½ sliced
½ head of broccoli
½ a bunch of fresh basil
30g hazelnuts
75ml extra virgin olive oil
sea salt and freshly ground black
    pepper

SERVES 2

Preheat the oven to 200°C/400°F/Gas Mark 6.

Tear off two large sheets of foil, lay a salmon fillet on each and place on a baking tray. Season well with salt and pepper.

Top each fillet with a slice of lemon. Wrap the foil tightly around the salmon and cook in the hot oven for around 12–15 minutes, or until cooked through.

Meanwhile, cut the broccoli into small florets and place in a food processor, along with the basil, hazelnuts, olive oil, lemon juice and a good pinch of salt and pepper.

Blitz for about a minute until you've achieved your desired consistency, adding splashes of water if needed, then tip into a bowl. Serve the salmon with your favourite side and a good helping of pesto, with an extra squeeze of lemon juice, if desired.

Lemon, Pineapple and Herb-Roasted Chicken with Greens

(DF) (GF) (V)

Another sweet and zesty way of pimping out your chicken for maximum taste.

100g fresh pineapple chunks
1 tbsp extra virgin olive oil
½ tsp dried oregano
2 lemons, 1½ juiced, ½ sliced
2 chicken thighs, skin on, bone in
200g Tenderstem broccoli
100g fresh baby spinach, finely chopped
sea salt and freshly ground black pepper

SERVES 2

Preheat the oven to 200°C/400°F/Gas Mark 6.

In a large bowl, mash the pineapple to a rough pulp, then add the olive oil, oregano and the juice from 1½ lemons.

Add the chicken, turn to coat and place in the fridge to marinate for about 15 minutes.

Put the marinated chicken into a roasting tray, skin side up. Add the lemon slices and cook in the hot oven for around 15 minutes.

To crisp up the skin, turn on the grill to medium-high and grill the chicken for 5 minutes, until the skin is nice and crispy.

Meanwhile, steam the broccoli for around 5–7 minutes, until tender. Season to taste with a little salt and pepper.

Serve the chicken with the chopped spinach, Tenderstem broccoli and the roasted lemon slices.

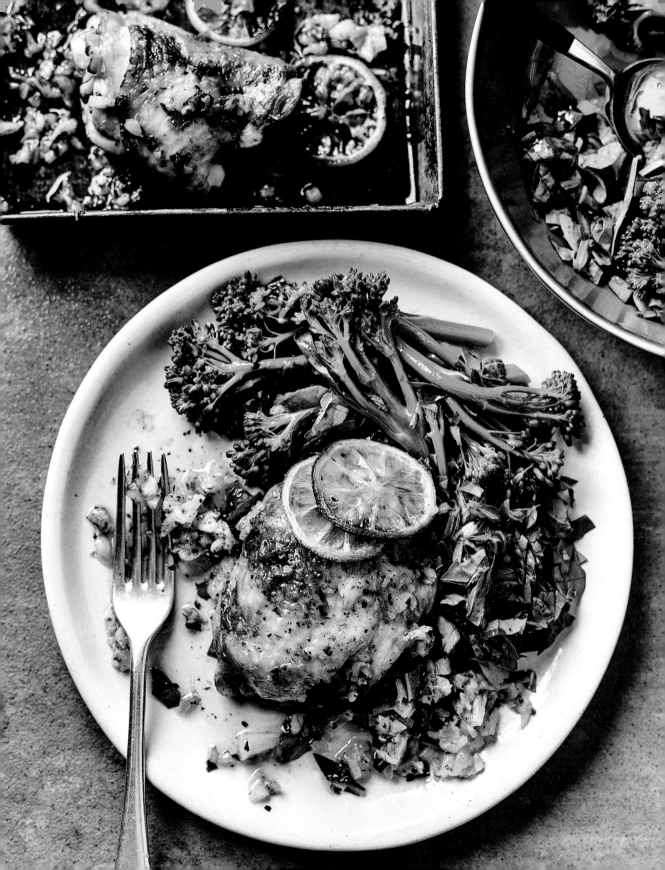

Thai Turkey Stir-fry with Chilli and Basil

DF GF

Simple dishes are often needed after busy days and this stir-fry requires minimum effort but delivers on taste. I use chilli in a lot of my dishes, as I love the added spice - but did you know that including chilli is also thought to help clear sinuses if you're suffering from a seasonal cold?

3 tsp coconut oil
400g skinless turkey breast, chopped
6 shallots, peeled, halved and sliced
4 garlic cloves, peeled and finely sliced
1 red chilli, finely sliced
1 lemongrass stalk
200g sugar snap peas
200g beansprouts
1 tbsp Thai fish sauce
1 lime, juiced
¼ of a bunch of fresh Thai basil leaves

SERVES 2

Heat half the coconut oil in a frying pan over a medium-high heat until melted and fry the turkey pieces for about 7 minutes until golden and cooked through, stirring often. Remove the turkey to a plate and return the pan to the heat.

Heat the rest of the oil in the pan until melted, add the shallots, garlic, chilli and lemongrass and fry for about 7 minutes, adding a splash of water if needed to stop it catching, stirring often. Add the sugar snap peas and beansprouts and cook for a further 5 minutes.

In a bowl, mix together the Thai fish sauce, lime juice and 2 tablespoons of water. Add to the pan along with the turkey, and continue to fry for another minute or so, until completely combined.

Serve scattered with the fresh Thai basil.

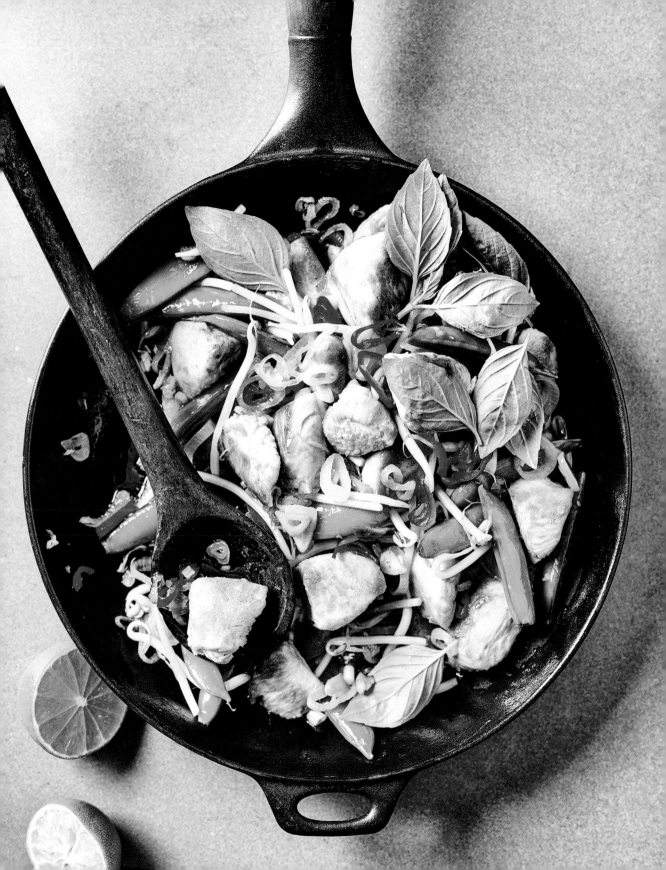

Citrus Roasted Root Veg with Gooey Goat's Cheese

GF V

If you fancy a meat-free meal, this delicious combination of starchy root vegetables and creamy goat's cheese is the one.

3 tbsp raspberry vinegar
1 tbsp extra virgin olive oil
1 tbsp honey
1 red chilli, halved, deseeded and diced
½ orange, zested and juiced
2 beetroots, trimmed, peeled and cut into 5mm thick slices
2 carrots, peeled and cut into 5cm batons
2 parsnips, peeled and cut into 5cm batons
1 red onion, peeled, halved and cut into wedges
2 x 30g rounds of goat's cheese
50g rocket
sea salt and freshly ground black pepper

SERVES 2

Preheat the oven to 200°C/400°F/Gas Mark 6.

In a bowl, mix the raspberry vinegar with the olive oil, honey, chilli, orange zest and juice. Season well and mix again until completely combined.

Tip the beetroot, carrot, parsnip and onion into a large roasting tray, drizzle with three-quarters of the dressing and toss so that the veggies are completely covered.

Roast in the hot oven for around 35–40 minutes.

Remove the tray of veggies from the oven, sit the individual goat's cheese rounds on top and put back into the oven to cook for a further 3 minutes.

Serve each individual goat's cheese round with half the veggies and a handful of rocket, and drizzle with the remaining dressing.

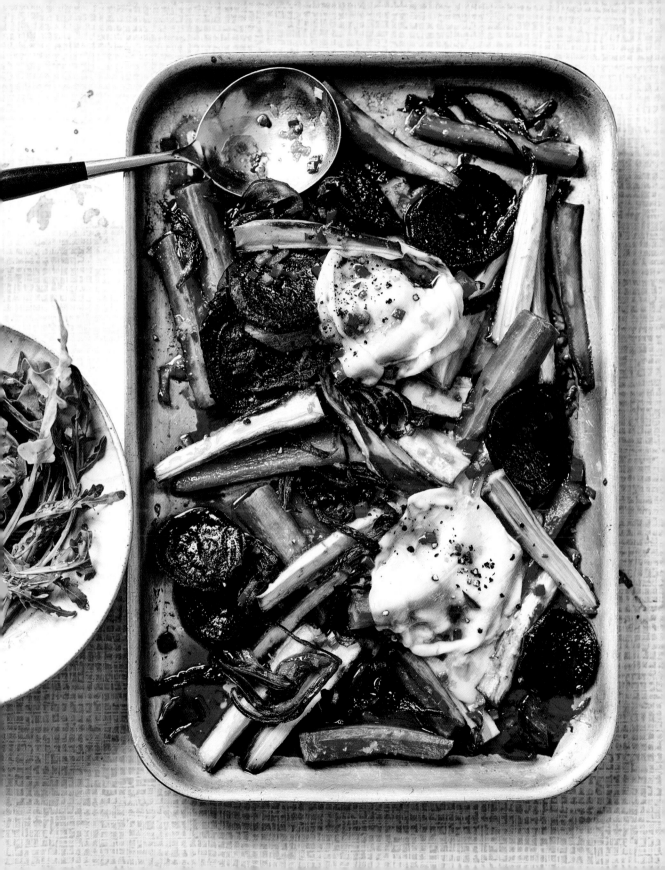

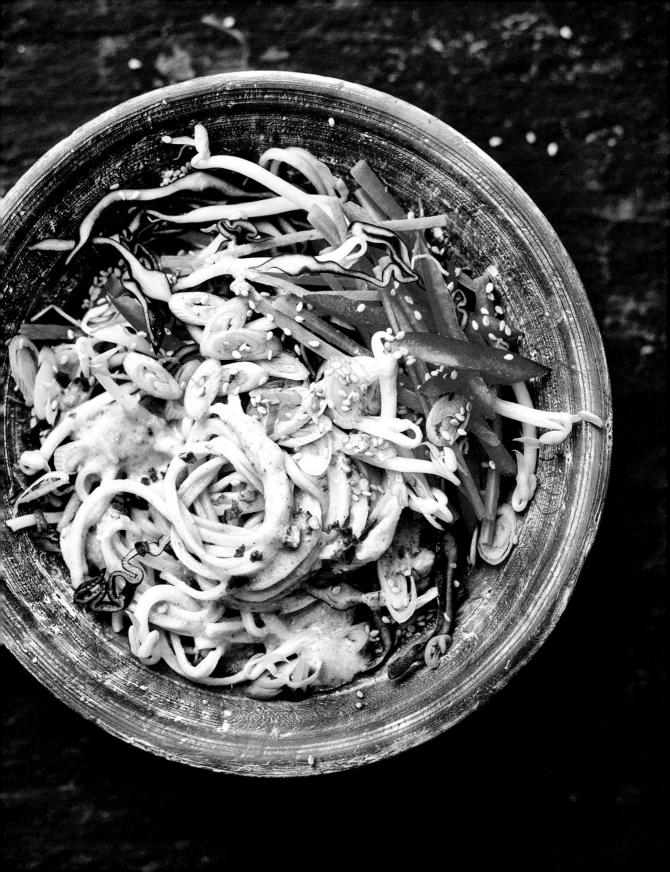

Asian-style Shredded Rainbow Veggie Noodle Salad

DF V

I'm always encouraging people to 'eat the rainbow', and this veggie salad allows just that!

100g wholewheat noodles
1 tsp sesame seeds
1 tbsp extra virgin olive oil
1 tbsp rice wine vinegar
1 tbsp peanut butter
1 lime, juiced
a pinch of chilli flakes
1 large carrot, peeled
1 red pepper, halved, deseeded and
 thinly sliced
¼ head of red cabbage, thinly sliced
50g beansprouts
1 spring onion, thinly sliced
sea salt

SERVES 2

Cook the noodles according to the packet instructions, then drain and rinse under cold water.

Place the sesame seeds in a small frying pan over a medium-high heat and toast until golden, shaking the pan often. Remove from the heat and set aside.

Mix the extra virgin olive oil with the rice wine vinegar, peanut butter and lime juice, 1 teaspoon of water, a pinch of chilli flakes and sea salt and stir to combine.

Use a julienne peeler to julienne the carrot, then tip into a large mixing bowl. Add the drained and cooled noodles, red pepper, red cabbage and beansprouts. Pour over the dressing and toss gently until completely coated.

Top with the toasted sesame seeds and sliced spring onion.

Quick Butter Bean Tagine with Herby Quinoa

With an extra-spicy kick, this is the perfect quick and simple lunch to throw together for minimum effort but maximum taste.

1 tbsp coconut oil

1 onion, peeled, halved and finely sliced

½ tsp ground cumin

½ tsp ground coriander

400g tinned butter beans, drained

200g tinned chopped tomatoes

1 red chilli, deseeded and finely sliced

50g quinoa, rinsed

a few sprigs of fresh coriander, leaves chopped

SERVES 1

Heat the coconut oil in a large frying pan over a medium heat until melted. Add the onion and fry for 5–7 minutes until softened.

Add the spices with a pinch of salt and pepper and stir to coat. Cook for a further 1–2 minutes, then add the butter beans, chopped tomatoes and chilli and bring to a gentle simmer. Simmer for 10–15 minutes until thickened, stirring occasionally and adding a splash of water if needed.

Meanwhile, place the quinoa in a saucepan, cover with cold salted water and place over a medium heat. Bring to the boil, reduce the heat to low and simmer for 15 minutes until cooked through, adding extra water if needed. Drain and tip into a bowl.

Serve the tagine on top of the quinoa, sprinkled with coriander.

Coriander and Chilli Grilled Chicken Fillets with Smashed Avocado and Wild Rice

DF GF

Packing in an excellent combination of protein, monounsaturated fats and carbohydrates, this covers all bases nutritionally, while also having a spicy kick to tingle your taste buds!

250g wild rice
½ avocado, peeled, halved and stoned
1 lime, juiced
½ tbsp fish sauce
1 large red chilli, halved and finely chopped (deseeded if you prefer a milder heat)
1 large garlic clove, peeled and minced
¼ of a bunch of fresh coriander, leaves chopped
5 spring onions, finely chopped
1 tbsp coconut oil
4 skinless boneless chicken thighs
sea salt and freshly ground black pepper

SERVES 2

Cook the rice according to the packet instructions. Mash the avocado with half the lime juice and season with salt and pepper.

In a small bowl, mix together the fish sauce, the remaining lime juice, chilli, garlic, coriander and spring onion.

Heat the coconut oil in a large frying pan over a high heat until melted. Season the chicken with salt and pepper and fry top side down for around 8 minutes until golden. Turn the thighs over, coat with two-thirds of the marinade and cook for a further 2 minutes, or until the chicken is cooked through.

Serve the chicken with the rice and avocado and drizzle over the remaining dressing.

Spiced Cod with Turmeric Roasted Cauliflower

GF

A diet high in cruciferous veggies such as cauliflower has been linked to a reduction in the risk of cancer. Cauliflower is also full of antioxidants and dietary fibre and is therefore a superfood that you should be including in your diet. Paired with some delicious baked fish and spices, this is a weeknight staple for me!

100g Greek yoghurt

1 small garlic clove, peeled and minced

2 sprigs each of fresh mint and coriander, leaves chopped

1 tsp turmeric, plus an extra pinch

¼ tsp ground cumin

2 large cod fillets

2 tbsp coconut oil

1 small cauliflower, cut into florets

sea salt and freshly ground black pepper

SERVES 2

In a bowl, mix the yoghurt and garlic with the chopped mint and coriander, a pinch of turmeric and the cumin until completely combined.

Add the cod, turn to coat and set aside to marinate.

Preheat the oven to 200°C/400°F/Gas Mark 6.

Put the coconut oil into a roasting tray and place in the hot oven until melted. Add the cauliflower, sprinkle over 1 teaspoon of turmeric, season with a little salt and pepper and toss to coat.

Roast in the hot oven for 40 minutes, adding the fish for the final 12 minutes, then serve.

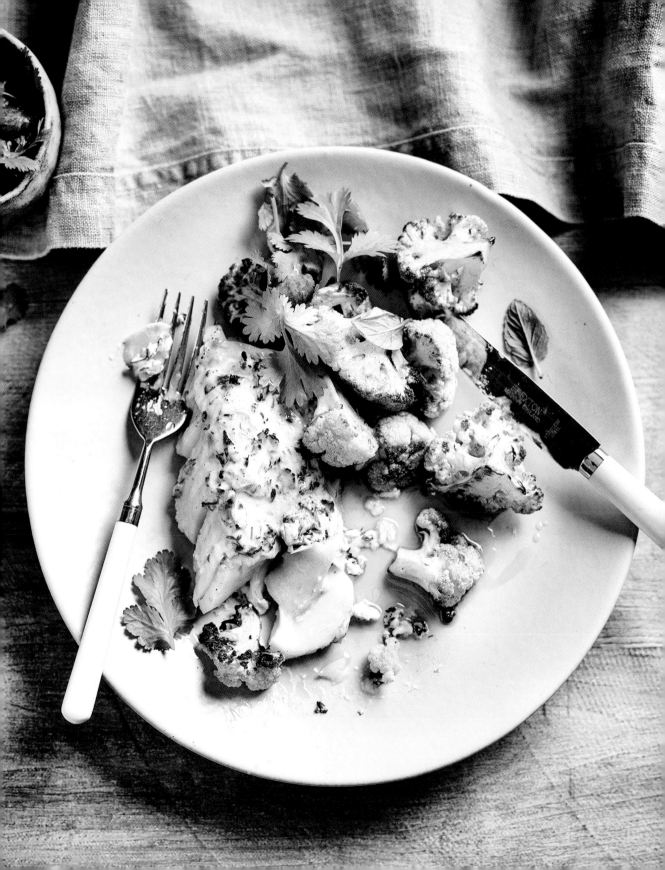

Cashew, Carrot, Pomegranate and Halloumi Salad

GF V

Halloumi is one of those foods that I could honestly eat every day! This dish pairs the salty taste of the cheese with the sweetness of pomegranate and it's a match made in heaven!

½ tbsp coconut oil
200g halloumi, sliced
20g cashew nuts
4 large carrots, peeled and coarsely grated
¼ of a bunch of fresh coriander, leaves chopped
50g pomegranate seeds

FOR THE DRESSING
3 tbsp tahini
1 tsp sumac
1½ limes, juiced
2 tbsp extra virgin olive oil
1½ tbsp apple cider vinegar
sea salt and freshly ground black pepper

SERVES 2

Heat the coconut oil in a frying pan over a medium-high heat until melted. Add the halloumi and fry on both sides until golden. Pat dry with some kitchen paper to remove any excess oil and set aside.

Carefully wipe the pan dry with kitchen paper and return to the heat. Add the cashew nuts and fry until lightly toasted, shaking the pan often, then remove from the heat and roughly chop.

Put the grated carrot, coriander, cashew nuts and pomegranate seeds into a large bowl.

Place all the dressing ingredients together in a jar with a pinch of salt and pepper, loosening with a dash of water if needed. Secure the lid and shake well until completely combined.

Pour the dressing over the bowl of carrot mixture, toss to coat and serve topped with the halloumi.

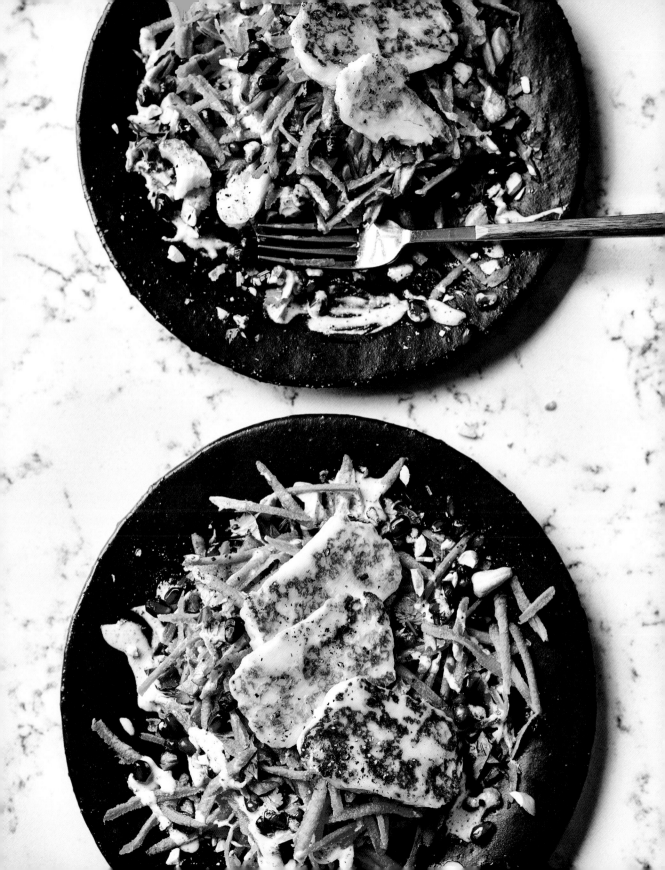

Mexican Quinoa Bowl

(DF) (GF) (V)

Perfect for post-workout yumminess, this nutrient-packed bowl will refuel energy levels and help towards repairing your muscles.

½ tbsp coconut oil

1 garlic clove, peeled and minced

1 green chilli, halved, deseeded and finely chopped (deseed if you prefer a milder heat)

½ vegetable stock cube

100g quinoa, rinsed

200g tinned kidney beans, drained

200g tinned chopped tomatoes

50g tinned sweetcorn, drained

½ tsp chilli powder

½ tsp ground cumin

1 avocado, peeled, halved, stoned and chopped

½ lime, juiced

a few sprigs of fresh coriander, leaves chopped

sea salt and freshly ground black pepper

SERVES 2

Heat the coconut oil in a large pan over a medium heat until melted. Add the garlic and green chilli and cook for about a minute, stirring often.

Dissolve the vegetable stock cube in 250ml boiling water and pour into the pan, then add the quinoa, kidney beans, tomatoes, sweetcorn, chilli powder and cumin and season well.

Bring to the boil, then cover, reduce the heat to medium-low and simmer for about 15 minutes, until the quinoa is cooked through, stirring occasionally.

Dish up into bowls and serve with the avocado, lime juice and coriander.

Beetroot and Feta Burgers

GF V

Tangy feta paired with the earthy taste of the beetroot makes these burgers deliciously moreish. Impress your guests by making them for a dinner party; I promise you, they won't disappoint!

3 beetroots, trimmed, peeled and grated
½ red onion, peeled and grated
1 large garlic clove, peeled and minced
100g rolled oats
2 tbsp extra virgin olive oil, plus extra for drizzling
1 free-range egg
75g feta, crumbled
¼ of a bunch of fresh mint, finely chopped
2 large tomatoes, sliced
50g lamb's lettuce
sea salt and freshly ground black pepper

SERVES 2

Put the grated beetroot, onion, garlic, rolled oats and olive oil into a large bowl and mix until fully combined.

In a separate bowl, whisk the egg. Add this to the grated veggie mixture with the feta and chopped mint. Season the mixture well with salt and pepper and place in the fridge for 30 minutes to allow the oats to soak up some of the moisture.

Preheat your oven to 180°C/350°F/Gas Mark 4 and line a baking tray with foil.

Using your hands, create four burger patties from the mixture. Place on the lined tray and cook in the hot oven for 13 minutes.

Remove the tray from the oven, lay the tomato slices around the burgers, season with salt and place back in the oven to cook for a further 7 minutes, until the burgers are cooked through

Serve the burgers on the lamb's lettuce with the roasted tomato slices and drizzle with olive oil.

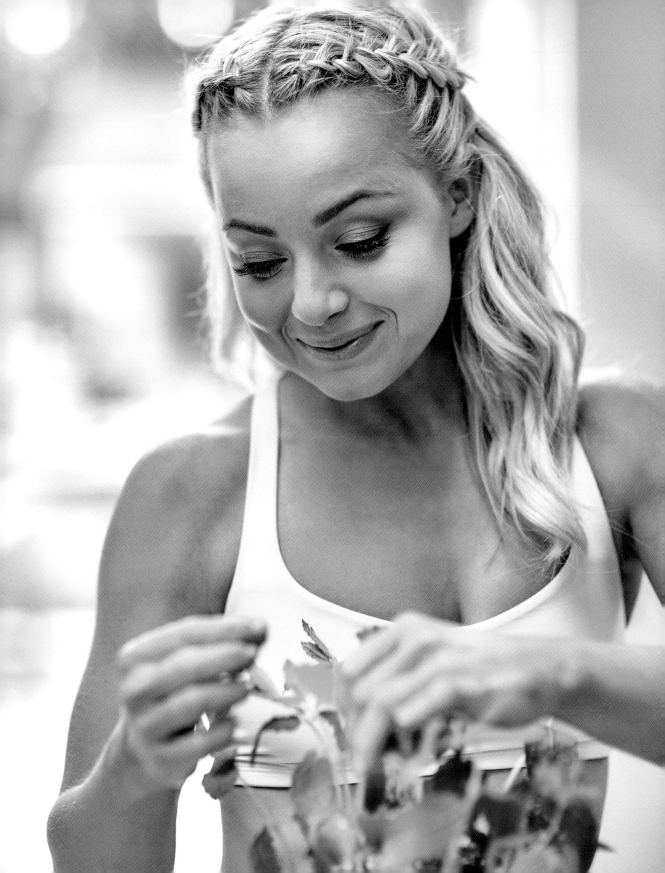

SNACKS

Raw Salted Caramel Slices

Seriously good snacking and so moreish, the natural sweetness of the Medjool dates means that these aren't as naughty as they taste.

200g Medjool dates, pitted
200g pecan nuts
60g desiccated coconut
2 tsp vanilla extract
1 tsp sea salt
1 tbsp date syrup
coconut oil, for greasing

MAKES 9

Tip the dates into a bowl, cover with boiling water and leave to soak for around 10 minutes, then drain.

Put the pecan nuts, desiccated coconut, vanilla extract, sea salt and date syrup into a food processor. Add the dates and blitz until smooth.

Grease an 18cm square baking tin with coconut oil and transfer the mixture into the tin, patting it down to flatten.

Place in the fridge for an hour to set, and then remove and slice into 9 squares.

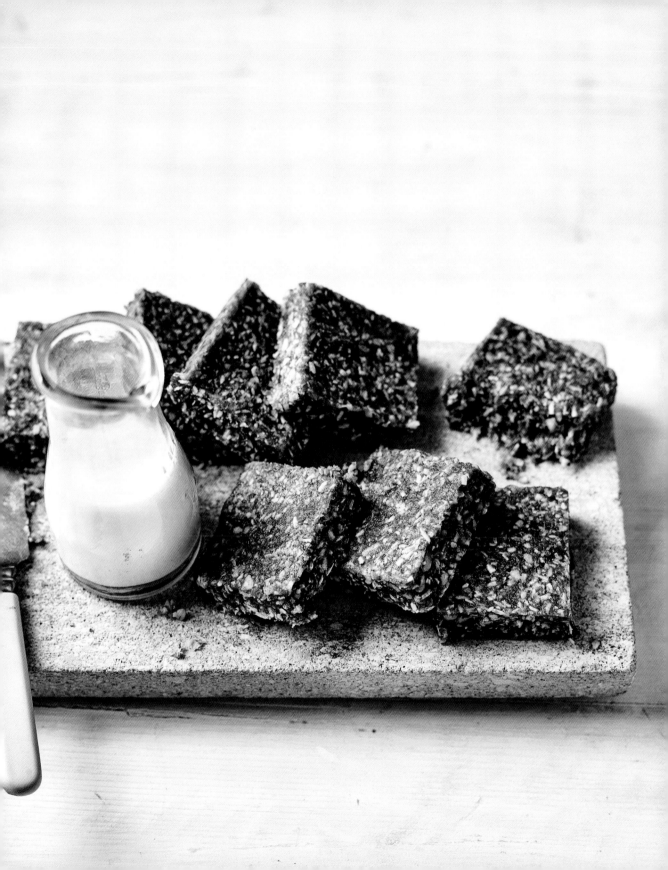

Brilliant Beetroot Energy Balls

(DF) (GF) (V)

Beetroots have long been hailed for their brilliant nutritional profile, providing an excellent source of the amino acid glutamine, folic acid and fibre. These quick and simple energy balls are therefore packed full of goodness, and are perfect to pop in a container for on-the-go fuel.
Pictured overleaf.

100g hazelnuts
1 large cooked beetroot, peeled and
    chopped (about 100g)
2 ripe bananas, peeled and chopped
225g rolled oats
2 tbsp maple syrup
1 tsp ground cinnamon
5 tbsp chia seeds

MAKES 12

Tip the hazelnuts into a dry frying pan. Place over a medium heat and toast until golden, shaking the pan often. Remove from the heat and leave to cool.

In a food processor, blitz the beetroot and bananas to a smooth purée. Add the oats, maple syrup, toasted hazelnuts and cinnamon and blitz again until the mixture forms a smooth paste. Place in the fridge to chill for 30 minutes.

Tip the chia seeds onto a plate and gently shake to evenly spread out. Line another plate with greaseproof paper.

Using your hands, take small amounts of the chilled mixture and roll it into balls before rolling in the chia seeds to coat. Place on the lined plate and chill in the fridge for about an hour. If not eating straight away, store in an airtight container in the fridge.

Vanilla Chickpea Energy Balls

DF GF V

Sweet and simple, the chickpeas in these energy balls provide a good source of protein - guaranteed to keep you full during busy days!
Pictured overleaf.

85g blanched almonds
400g tin of chickpeas, drained
    and rinsed
250g peanut butter
2 tbsp maple syrup
1 tsp vanilla extract

MAKES 30

Line a small baking tray with greaseproof paper.

Blitz the almonds in a food processor to a flour-like consistency. Add the chickpeas and blitz until fully broken down.

Add the peanut butter, maple syrup and vanilla extract and blitz until smooth.

Tip the mixture out and, using your hands, roll it into small balls and place on the lined baking tray. Place in the freezer to set for at least 25 minutes. If not eating straight away, store in an airtight container in the fridge.

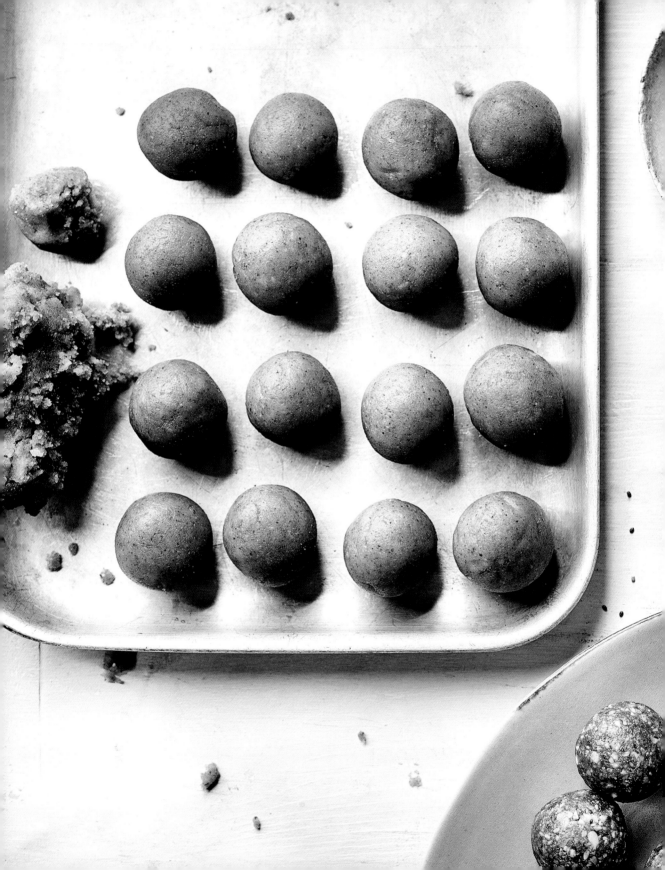

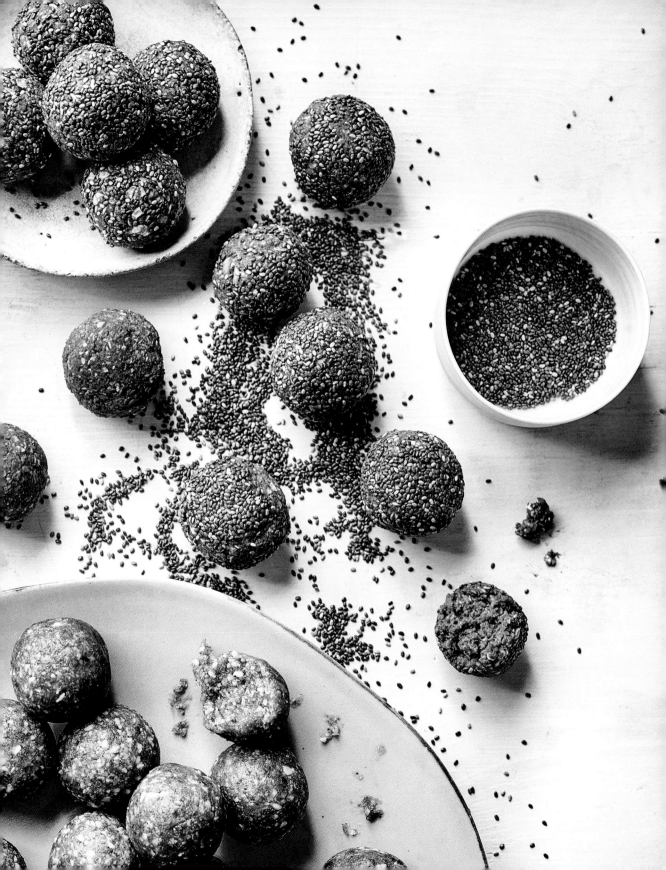

Date and Almond Energy Balls

(DF) (GF) (V)

These energy balls get their natural sweetness from the delicious dates, which are also an excellent source of fibre! With no added refined sugars, these are definitely the perfect healthy simple swap. Pictured on pages 160–161.

225g Medjool dates, pitted
170g blanched almonds
125g almond butter
1 tsp vanilla extract
1 tsp ground cinnamon
1 tbsp unsweetened almond milk
    (optional)

MAKES 12

Tip the dates into a bowl, cover with boiling water and leave to soak for around 10 minutes, then drain. Line a plate with greaseproof paper.

Blitz the almonds in a food processor to a flour-like consistency.

Add the dates, almond butter, vanilla extract and cinnamon and blitz until the mixture starts to come together – if it helps, add 1 tablespoon of almond milk. You may need to use a spatula to scrape the sides down a few times so that the dates fully combine.

Tip the mixture out and, using your hands, roll it into small balls and place on the lined plate. Place in the fridge for around 30 minutes. If not eating straight away, store in an airtight container in the fridge.

Super Simple Banana and Blueberry Loaf

DF GF V

Perfect for weekend baking, this loaf is simple yet scrumptious and makes the perfect snack to see you through the week.

3 tbsp coconut oil, plus extra
    for greasing
3 very ripe bananas, peeled
3 free-range eggs
3 tbsp maple syrup
½ tsp vanilla extract
180g almond flour
1 tsp baking powder
150g blueberries

MAKES A 450g (1LB) LOAF

Preheat the oven to 180°C/350°F/Gas Mark 4. Grease a 450g (1LB) loaf tin with coconut oil and line with greaseproof paper. Put the coconut oil into a small bowl and heat in the microwave until melted.

In a mixing bowl, use a fork to mash the bananas to a smooth pulp. Crack in the eggs, then pour in the melted coconut oil, maple syrup and vanilla extract and mix until fully combined.

Whisk in the almond flour and baking powder until well combined (it is best to use an electric whisk for this). Finally, fold in most of the blueberries, saving a small handful to place on top.

Pour the mixture into the lined tin, push the reserved blueberries into the top and bake in the hot oven for 50–60 minutes or until cooked through and a knife inserted comes out clean.

Super Strawberry Crush Smoothie

Deliciously light and fresh, the hint of mint in this smoothie gives it the perfect summer twist – great for warm summer days!

½ frozen banana, peeled and chopped
8 large strawberries, hulled
1 tbsp Greek yoghurt
3 ice cubes
100ml unsweetened almond milk
a few fresh mint leaves

SERVES 1

Place all the ingredients in a blender, blitz until thick and creamy and serve.

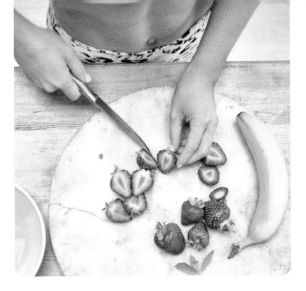
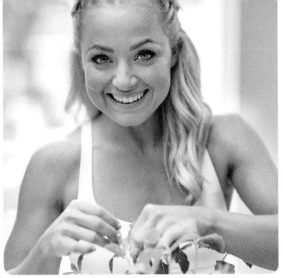
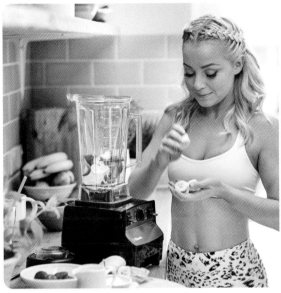
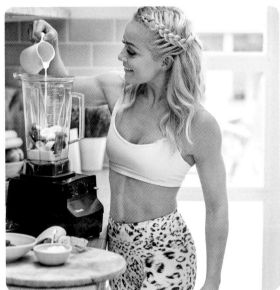
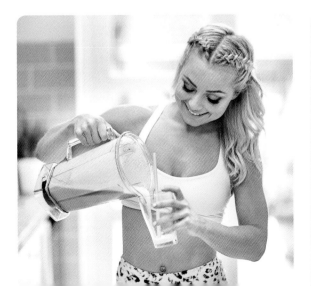
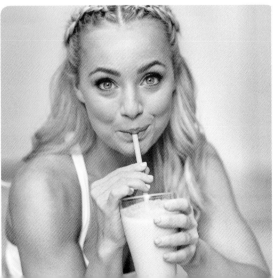

Cashew and Kale Crisps

DF GF V

Loaded with flavour, these spiced crisps are the perfect simple swap to snack on.

3 tbsp cashew nuts
2 tbsp sunflower seeds
½ tsp sea salt
a pinch of paprika
1 small garlic clove, peeled
¼ lemon, juiced
3 large handfuls of kale, large stems removed (about 200g)

Tip the cashews into a bowl, cover with about 200ml boiling water and leave to soak for at least 1 hour, then drain, reserving 5–6 tablespoons of the soaking water.

In a small food processor, place the sunflower seeds, cashew nuts, reserved soaking water, sea salt, paprika, garlic and lemon juice, and blitz until smooth and creamy.

Preheat the oven to 180°C/350°F/Gas Mark 4.

Put the kale into a large mixing bowl, pour over the cashew cream, then, using your hands, toss the kale until it is completely covered.

Spread the kale on two baking trays in a single layer and cook in the hot oven for around 7–10 minutes until crispy. Transfer to a wire rack to cool.

Super Simple Beetroot Crisps

DF **GF** **V**

These crisps are the perfect snack – the prep is easy and they store well, too. Try serving them to friends as a nibble before dinner!

2 tbsp coconut oil
4 medium beetroots, trimmed
½ tsp sea salt

Preheat the oven to 200°C/400°F/Gas Mark 6. Line two large baking trays with greaseproof paper.

Put the coconut oil into a small bowl and heat in the microwave until melted.

Using a very sharp knife, carefully slice the beetroots into very thin slices. You can also do this using a mandolin or the slicing attachment of a food processor.

Put the beetroot slices into a bowl, pour over the melted coconut oil, sprinkle over the salt and toss until coated.

Spread the slices on the two lined baking trays, making sure they don't overlap. Cook in the hot oven for around 10–15 minutes, then turn the slices over and bake for a further 5 minutes. Remove from the oven and transfer to a wire rack to cool.

Spicy Oven-roasted Chickpeas

(DF) (GF) (V)

Free of refined sugar and full of flavour, these roasted chickpeas are an excellent source of protein, and perfect for snacking on the go.

2 tbsp coconut oil
1 tsp ground cumin
1 tsp chilli powder
½ tsp cayenne pepper
½ tsp sea salt flakes
400g tinned chickpeas, drained and patted dry

Preheat the oven to 200°C/400°F/Gas Mark 6. Line a baking tray with greaseproof paper. Put the coconut oil into a large bowl and heat in the microwave until melted.

Stir the spices and salt into the melted coconut oil, add the chickpeas and stir to fully coat.

Tip the chickpeas onto the lined baking tray, spread out evenly and roast in the hot oven for around 30–35 minutes, until crisp.

Remove from the oven and transfer to a wire rack to cool.

Blueberry Flapjacks

GF V

A childhood favourite of mine, these are a simple alternative to shop-bought, sugar-loaded snack bars.

100g butter, plus extra
   for greasing
200g rolled oats
100g ground almonds
1 tsp ground cinnamon
100g fresh blueberries
2 tbsp maple syrup

MAKES 8

Preheat the oven to 200°C/400°F/Gas Mark 6. Grease a 30cm x 15cm baking tin and line with greaseproof paper.

In a mixing bowl, combine the oats and ground almonds with the cinnamon and stir in the blueberries.

Melt the butter in a small pan over a low heat. As the butter begins to melt, add the maple syrup, then pour into the oat mixture and stir to combine.

Transfer the mixture into the lined baking tin and use the back of a wooden spoon to firmly press it down. Bake in the hot oven for around 20 minutes, or until golden.

Transfer to a wire rack to cool before cutting into individual squares. Store in an airtight container.

Dark Chocolate Orange Cookies

(DF) (GF) (V)

This is a seriously good combo, loaded into a cookie. So. Much. YUM!

50g rolled oats
40g desiccated coconut
125g Medjool dates, pitted
70g sunflower seeds
45g unsalted butter, softened
½ orange, juiced and zested
a small handful of dairy-free dark
    chocolate chips

MAKES 12–14

Blitz the oats, desiccated coconut, dates and sunflower seeds in a food processor for about 1 minute until completely broken down and crumb-like.

Add the butter, orange zest and juice and chocolate chips. Further blitz until the mixture comes together to form a dough.

Tip the mixture out onto a clean surface and roll it into a log shape about 5cm in diameter. Wrap in cling film and place in the freezer to firm up for around 20 minutes.

Preheat the oven to 170°C/325°F/Gas Mark 3 and line a baking tray with greaseproof paper.

Once firmed up, remove the cookie dough from the freezer, remove the cling film and slice the dough into rounds slightly less than 1cm thick with a serrated knife.

Place the rounds on the lined baking tray and cook in the hot oven for around 15 minutes or until golden, then transfer to a wire rack to cool.

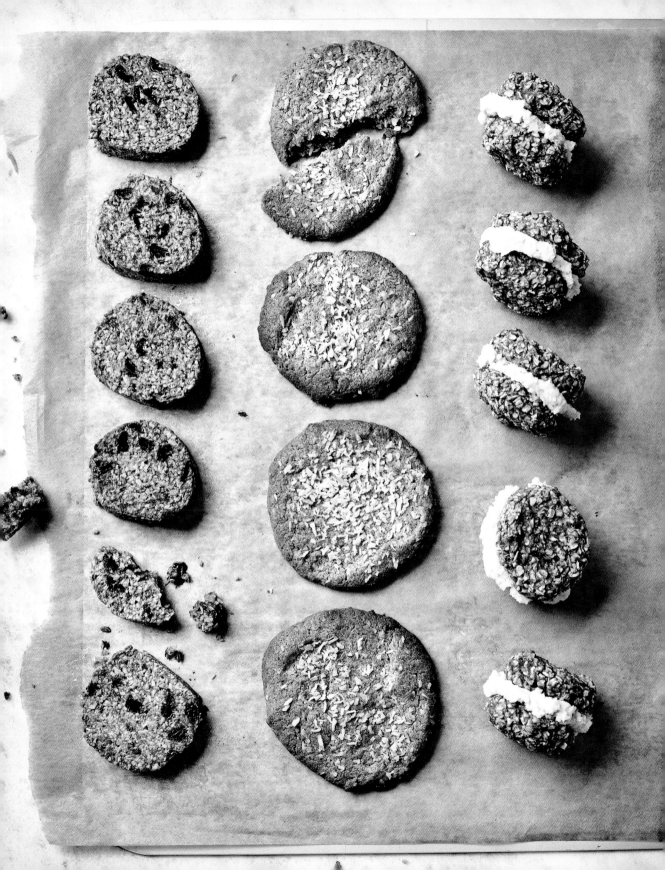

Coconut and Almond Butter Cookies

DF GF V

These delicious treats packed with healthy fats couldn't be simpler to make and will trump any processed shop-bought version! Pictured on page 171

55g coconut oil
250g almond butter
2 ½ tbsp maple syrup
1 tsp vanilla extract
1 tsp ground cinnamon
1 free-range egg
1 tbsp coconut flour
20g desiccated coconut

MAKES 12–14

Put the coconut oil into a small bowl and heat in the microwave until melted, then pour into a mixing bowl. Add the almond butter, maple syrup, vanilla extract and cinnamon. Crack in the egg and mix until completely combined.

Next, add the coconut flour and half the desiccated coconut. Stir to combine, then place in the fridge to chill for at least 30 minutes. If you are short of time, place in the freezer for 15 minutes instead.

Preheat the oven to 170°C/325°F/Gas Mark 3.

Line two baking trays with greaseproof paper. Spoon the mixture into cookie shapes on the trays and gently flatten each with the back of a spoon. Sprinkle with the remaining desiccated coconut.

Cook in the hot oven for 15 minutes, or until golden, then transfer to a wire rack to cool.

Oatmeal Cookie Sandwiches with Coconut and Lemon Cashew Cream

My sweet and light twist on a stuffed cookie – impress your friends with these zesty treats!
Pictured on page 171

100g cashew nuts
4 very ripe bananas, peeled and chopped
150g rolled oats
1 tsp ground cinnamon
50g desiccated coconut
1 lemon, zested
1 tbsp maple syrup
5 tbsp coconut milk

MAKES 5

Put the cashew nuts into a bowl, cover with warm water and leave to soak overnight.

Preheat the oven to 180°C/350°F/Gas Mark 4. Line two baking trays with greaseproof paper.

In a mixing bowl, mash the bananas into a smooth pulp using a fork. Mix in the oats and cinnamon and leave to stand for around 5 minutes for the oats to soften.

Meanwhile, drain the cashews and put into a food processor with the desiccated coconut, lemon zest, maple syrup and coconut milk and blitz until smooth. Tip the mixture into a sealable container and place in the fridge to chill.

Using your hands, form the banana and oat mixture into 10 cookie-sized balls. Place on the lined trays and gently flatten each with a fork until 1cm thick. Cook in the hot oven for around 13 minutes or until golden, then transfer to a wire rack to cool.

Once cooled, spread a layer of the cashew cream on one cookie, then sandwich another on top. Repeat with the remaining cookies.

Kale, Avocado and Citrus Smoothie

This zesty smoothie gets its creaminess from the avocado and Greek yoghurt combination. Perfect for post-workout refuelling or a quick on-the-go breakfast!

1 frozen banana, peeled and chopped
1 tbsp Greek yoghurt
1 large handful of kale, any large stems removed
½ ripe avocado, peeled and stoned
1 lime, zested and ½ juiced
200ml unsweetened almond milk

SERVES 1

Put all the ingredients into a blender, blitz until smooth and serve.

Mango and Lime 'Slushie'

The old favourite cinema treat just got a healthy twist – zesty and light, this is a summer special that you have to try!

100g mango, peeled, halved, stoned and frozen
1 tbsp Greek yoghurt
5 ice cubes
150ml unsweetened almond milk
½ lime, juiced
3 fresh mint leaves

SERVES 2

Put all the ingredients into a blender, blitz until smooth and serve.

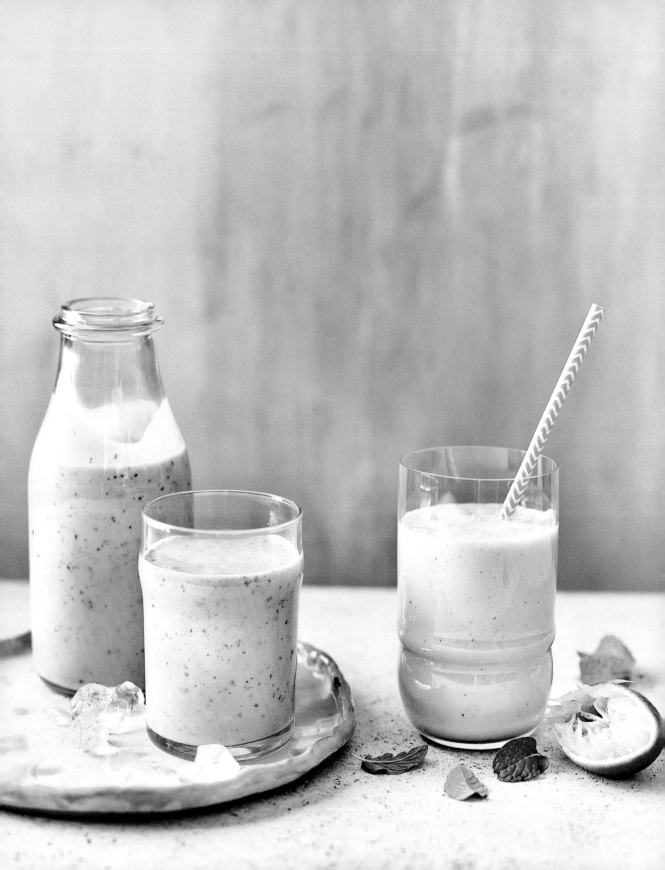

Chocolate Chia Smoothie

(DF) (GF) (V)

Cacao has powerful antioxidant effects, so this smoothie not only tastes great, but delivers nutritionally, too.

½ banana, peeled, chopped
    and frozen
1 tbsp cacao powder
½ tbsp chia seeds
2 Medjool dates, pitted
a large handful of fresh spinach
200ml unsweetened almond milk

SERVES 1

Put all the ingredients into a blender, blitz until smooth and serve.

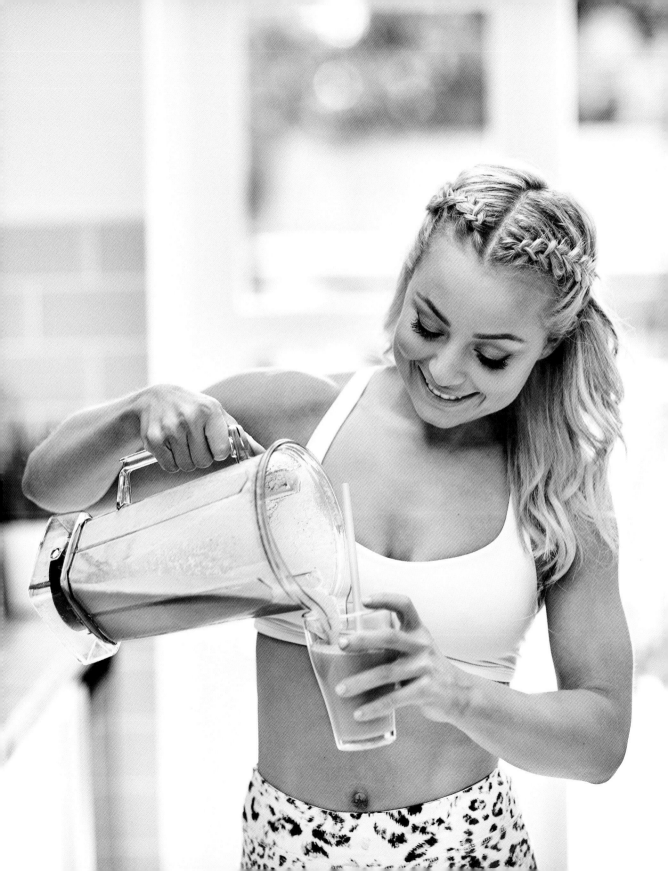

Homemade Blackberry Chia Jam with Greek Yoghurt

GF **V**

This jam couldn't be simpler to make, and is an excellent alternative to shop-bought varieties. Chia seeds are also a natural source of calcium, iron and magnesium, needed for healthy bones, teeth and immune system.

½ tsp coconut oil
450g blackberries
2 tbsp maple syrup
2 tbsp chia seeds
½ tsp vanilla extract
150g Greek yoghurt (per serving)

MAKES ABOUT 375g JAM

Heat the coconut oil in a saucepan over a medium-high heat until melted. Add the blackberries and cook for a few minutes until they come to a low boil, stirring frequently.

Reduce the heat to low and simmer for around 10 minutes until the blackberries have completely softened, stirring occasionally.

Using a fork, gently mash the blackberries to a smooth pulp, then stir in the maple syrup and chia seeds and cook for a further 5–7 minutes until thickened.

Remove from the heat, stir in the vanilla extract and set aside to cool to room temperature.

Once cooled, serve over Greek yoghurt and store the remaining jam in an airtight container in the fridge.

Chewy Coconut, Cashew and Chia Bars

(DF) (GF) (V)

Some of my favourite flavours rolled into a delicious snack bar, these are another perfect weekend baking treat that means you've got snacks to grab on those busy weekdays!

200g cashew nuts
coconut oil, for greasing
110g date syrup
25g almond flour
1 tbsp almond butter
a pinch of sea salt
5 Medjool dates, pitted and chopped
60g desiccated coconut
1 tbsp chia seeds

MAKES 10

Put the cashew nuts into a bowl, cover with warm water and leave to soak for 2 hours.

Preheat the oven to 170°C/325°F/Gas Mark 3. Grease a 20cm baking tin with coconut oil and line with greaseproof paper.

In a mixing bowl, combine the date syrup, almond flour and almond butter with a pinch of sea salt. Drain the cashew nuts and gently fold into the mixture along with the dates, desiccated coconut and chia seeds and mix until fully combined.

Transfer the mixture into the lined baking tin and use the back of a wooden spoon to firmly press it down. You want to pack it down as tight as possible.

Bake in the hot oven for around 20 minutes, or until golden. Remove and leave to cool in the tin, before transferring to a wire rack to cool for around 1 hour. Place in the fridge to chill for another hour, then slice into 10 and store in an airtight container.

PLATES

When trying to get healthy and make that all-important change, we often forget it is about taking small steps in the right direction, rather than trying to do it all at once.

We often see beautiful recipes on the pages of cookbooks and wonder how we will ever recreate that in real life. Often the food looks perfect, not a stray basil leaf out of place, and it can be intimidating.

This is something I have tried to address ever since I started posting my food on Instagram. One of my main aims was always to show the reality of my cooking and the 'realness' of my food. It can be messy and it is always real – I don't style my plates to look picture perfect, as that isn't how I live. Particularly having been on the road during my *Annie* tour, so much of what I ate was cooked in a kitchen that wasn't my own, using what I could find from local supermarkets and eaten in a hurry – it certainly didn't look photo-shoot ready.

This section will show you in a bit more detail how and why I build my meals the way I do, so that you can be equipped with the knowledge you need for your day-to-day eating. The key is to show you how I eat and why I group foods in a certain way at different times of the day.

We scroll through Instagram and see beautiful meals, but without any explanation of what is on the plate. With so much information out there, and so many conflicting messages, it can be confusing. What I have done here is broken it down so that you understand better why these foods are in my everyday diet, what I think they do to my body and why.

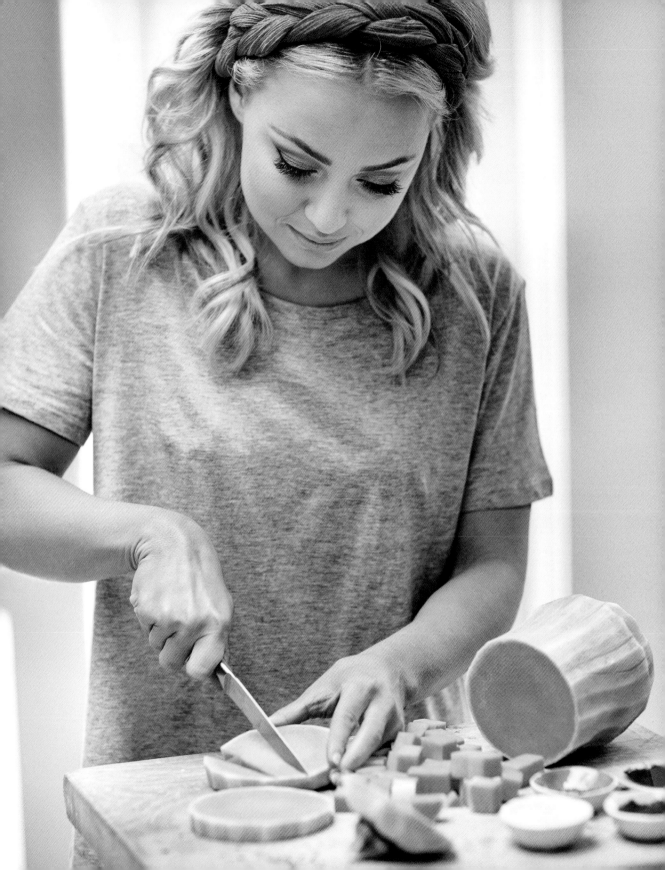

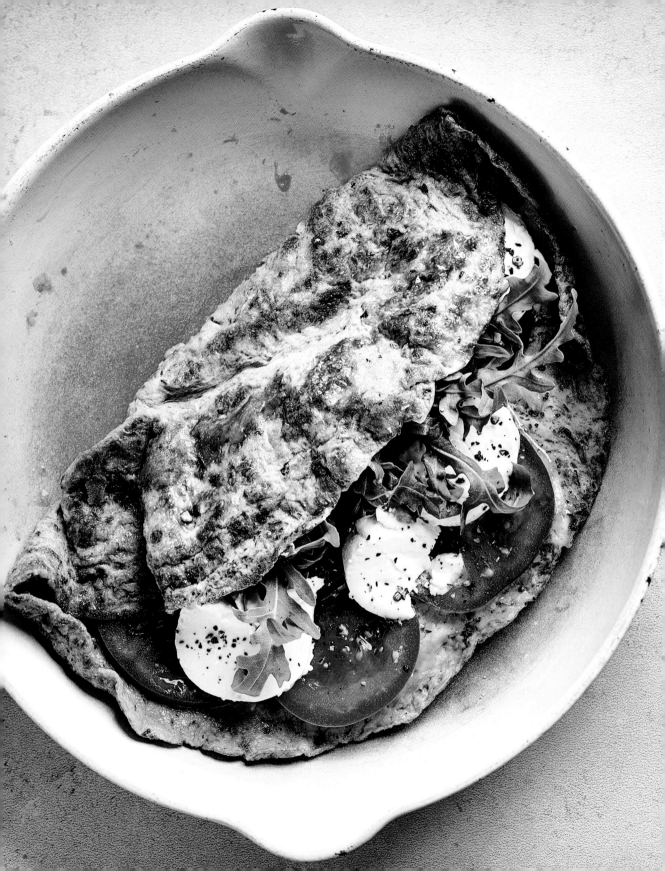

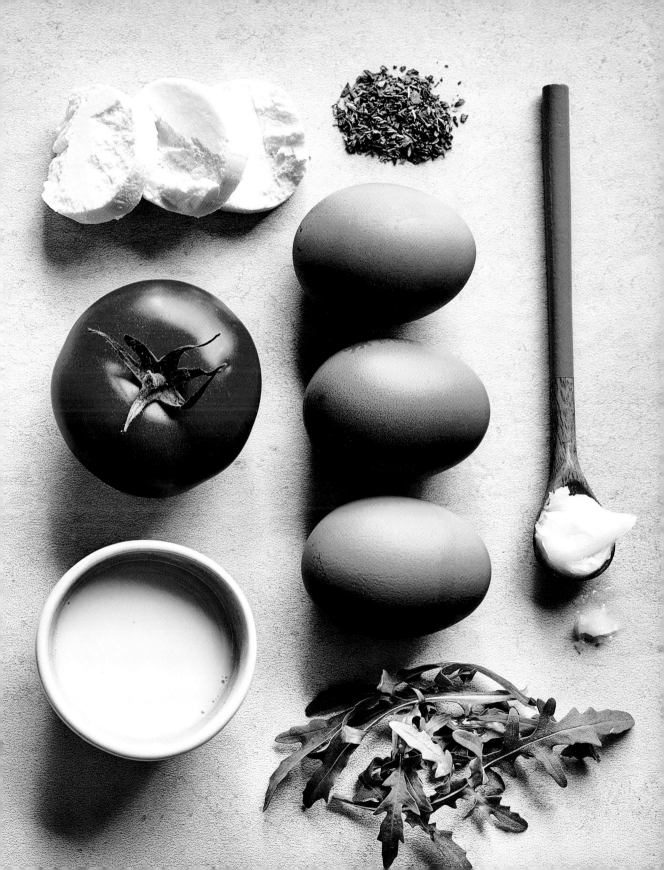

Rest-day plate:
Gooey Goat's Cheese, Tomato and Rocket Omelette

GF V

Nothing beats gooey cheese in my opinion, and this omelette will certainly deliver on taste and texture. Packed full of protein, this is the perfect indulgence for a rest day.

3 free-range eggs
1 tbsp unsweetened almond milk
¼ tsp dried mixed herbs
1 tsp coconut oil
1 small ripe tomato, thinly sliced
40g goat's cheese, thinly sliced
a small handful of rocket
sea salt and freshly ground black pepper

SERVES 1

Crack the eggs into a large bowl and whisk until fully combined. Add the almond milk, herbs and a pinch of salt and pepper and whisk for a further few seconds.

Heat the coconut oil in a large non-stick frying pan over a medium-low heat until melted. Pour in the egg mixture and leave to cook for a few minutes until the base begins to set.

Evenly scatter over the tomato and goat's cheese.

Once the top of the omelette has almost set, scatter over the rocket, fold to seal, then serve.

Why this works

This for me is a perfect rest-day treat breakfast. On rest days I maintain the same calorie intake as on days when I exercise. Your body still needs food to promote recovery from a week of training, even on your days off, so there should be no restriction or avoiding certain foods on a rest day!

1. Protein

Both eggs and goat's cheese are an excellent source of protein – three whole eggs provide around 18g of good-quality protein, while 40g of goat's cheese provides around 8g of protein – so this omelette ensures that you are kept satiated throughout the morning.

2. Micronutrients

I often like to include leafy greens in my omelettes and rocket is one of my favourites. With a peppery, tangy flavour, rocket is rich in phytochemicals, which have been shown to potentially reduce the risk of some cancers. It is also an excellent source of vitamins A and K, and provides dietary fibre.

More rest-day breakfast ideas:

Mushroom, Spinach and Feta Omelette (see recipe, page 58)

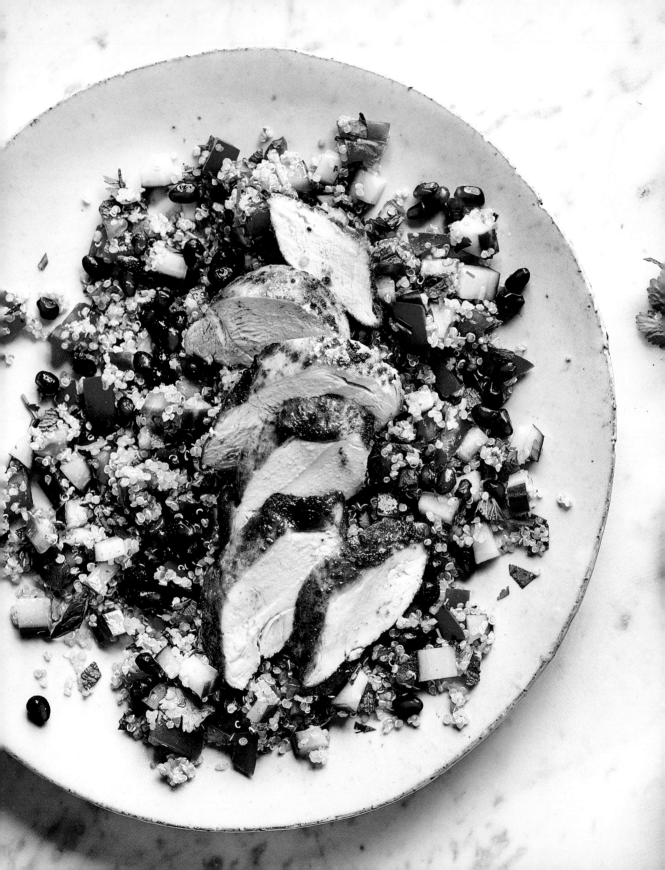

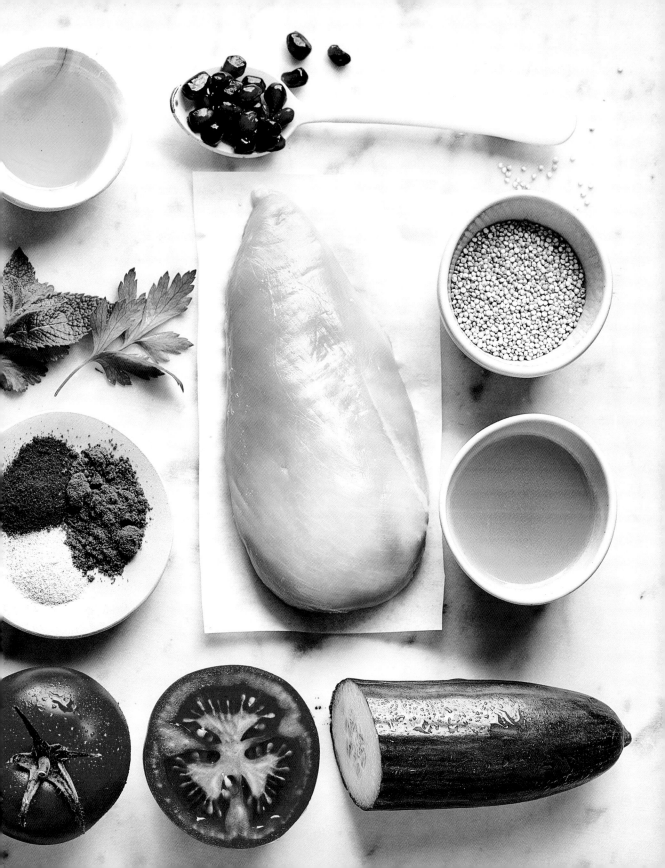

Rest-day dinner plate:
Spiced Roast Chicken with Quinoa Tabbouleh

The simple flavours and textures of this quinoa tabbouleh make it a firm favourite of mine, and always reminds me of holidays abroad.

¼ tsp paprika

¼ tsp ground cumin

a pinch of garlic salt

1 tbsp olive oil

2 large skinless, boneless chicken breasts

1 vegetable stock cube

100g quinoa, rinsed

½ cucumber, cut into small chunks

2 tomatoes, cut into small chunks

a few sprigs each of fresh mint, coriander and flat-leaf parsley, leaves finely chopped

50g pomegranate seeds

SERVES 2

Put the paprika, cumin, garlic salt and olive oil into a bowl. Add the chicken and turn to coat. Set aside to marinate for around 15 minutes.

Dissolve the vegetable stock cube in 600ml boiling water. Place the quinoa in a saucepan, cover with the stock and place over a medium heat. Bring to the boil, reduce the heat to low and simmer for 15 minutes until cooked through, adding extra water of needed. Drain and tip into a bowl.

Preheat the grill to medium. Line a baking sheet with foil.

Place the marinated chicken on the lined baking sheet and cook under the hot grill for 10 minutes, or until completely cooked through, turning halfway through. Then remove and slice. Meanwhile, stir the chopped cucumber, tomatoes, herbs and pomegranate seeds through the quinoa and serve topped with the sliced chicken.

Why this works

I'm one of those people who probably feels more hungry on their rest day than on the day that they train! This rest-day dinner plate is packed full of protein to promote and aid recovery, and paired with a slow-releasing carbohydrate, it will keep you feel satiated throughout the evening, too!

1. Protein

Both chicken and quinoa are good-quality sources of protein, making this an excellent meal to finish the day with!

2. Fats

This recipe includes olive oil, which is an excellent source of healthy mono-unsaturated fats. Research shows that consuming olive oil in your diet can help reduce the risk of hypertension; it also has anti-inflammatory properties and helps to lower LDL or bad cholesterol.

3. Carbohydrates

Quinoa is a slow-releasing carbohydrate, providing a steady release of energy into the body. Consuming carbs in the evening shouldn't be something that instils you with fear. Carbohydrates can actually help the release of serotonin, a hormone that is involved in helping you to feel sleepy!

4. Micronutrients

Pomegranate seeds are good sources of vitamins C and K and also provide dietary fibre.

More rest-day dinner ideas:

Thai-style Turkey Burgers (see recipe, page 97) or Harissa and Lime Salmon Parcels with Coconut Rice (see recipe, page 131).

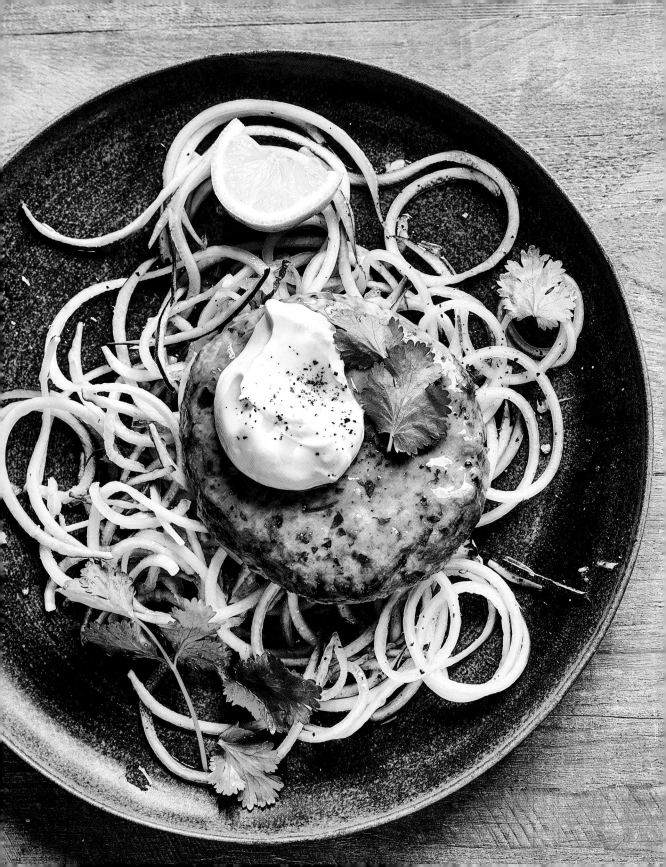

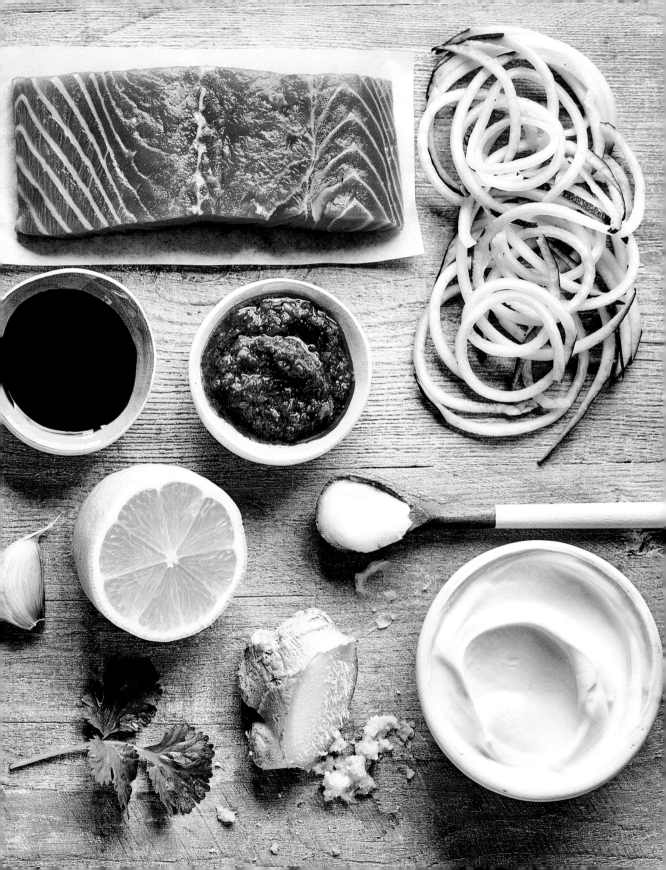

Lunch-on-the-go plate:
Spicy Salmon Burgers with Courgetti

A flavoursome twist on a classic, this low-carb lunch is brilliant for on-the-go fuel.

½ tsp coconut oil, for greasing

2 skinless salmon fillets

1 tbsp Thai red curry paste

a small chunk of ginger, peeled and grated

½ tsp soy sauce

¼ of a bunch of fresh coriander, leaves chopped

4 tbsp Greek yoghurt

1 small garlic clove, peeled and minced

½ lemon, juiced

2 large courgettes, trimmed

extra virgin olive oil, for drizzling

sea salt and freshly ground black pepper

SERVES 2

Preheat the oven to 200°C/400°F/Gas Mark 6. Line a baking tray with foil and grease with coconut oil.

Cut the salmon into chunks, place in a food processor with the red curry paste, ginger, soy sauce and chopped coriander and blitz until roughly minced.

Using your hands, shape the mixture into two burger patties and place on the lined baking tray. The burgers will seem quite soft, but they will firm up while cooking. Cook the burgers in the hot oven for 10 minutes or until cooked through.

Meanwhile, mix the Greek yoghurt with the garlic, half the lemon juice and a good pinch of salt and black pepper.

Use a spiralizer or julienne peeler to create courgetti or use a vegetable peeler to peel the courgettes into long ribbons, avoiding the seeds. Divide between two sealable containers – you can steam the courgetti for a couple of minutes first, if you prefer.

Place the cooked salmon burgers on top of the courgetti and top each burger with a tablespoon of the Greek yoghurt mixture. Drizzle over the remaining lemon juice and a little extra virgin olive oil and season with a pinch of sea salt and black pepper.

Why this works

I find these salmon burgers are the perfect meal prep. Paired with super-simple courgetti, it's simply a case of popping them into a sealable container and grabbing them when you need them. Packed full of essential healthy fats and protein, this is some serious food for busy days.

1. Protein

This meal has two main sources of protein: the salmon and the Greek yoghurt. With an average salmon fillet providing over 30g of protein, the fish is a tasty component of this meal and ensures that you stay feeling full while on the go.

3. Micronutrients

This recipe is full of dietary fibre from the courgette, and is also packed with micronutrients from the coriander, ginger and fresh lemon juice. Coriander is abundant in antioxidants.

2. Fats

Salmon champions two excellent sources of healthy fats, providing essential omega-3 fatty acids, while Greek yoghurt is a good source of probiotics that improve gut health (look out for good-quality yoghurt which contains probiotics). Drizzling this dish with a dash of olive oil will add extra healthy monounsaturated fats to your daily intake.

More lunch-on-the-go ideas:

Salmon, Seeds, Avocado and Dill (see recipe, page 90), Shredded Sprout, Bacon and Almond Salad (see recipe, page 95) or Souper Simple Broccoli Soup (see recipe, page 98)

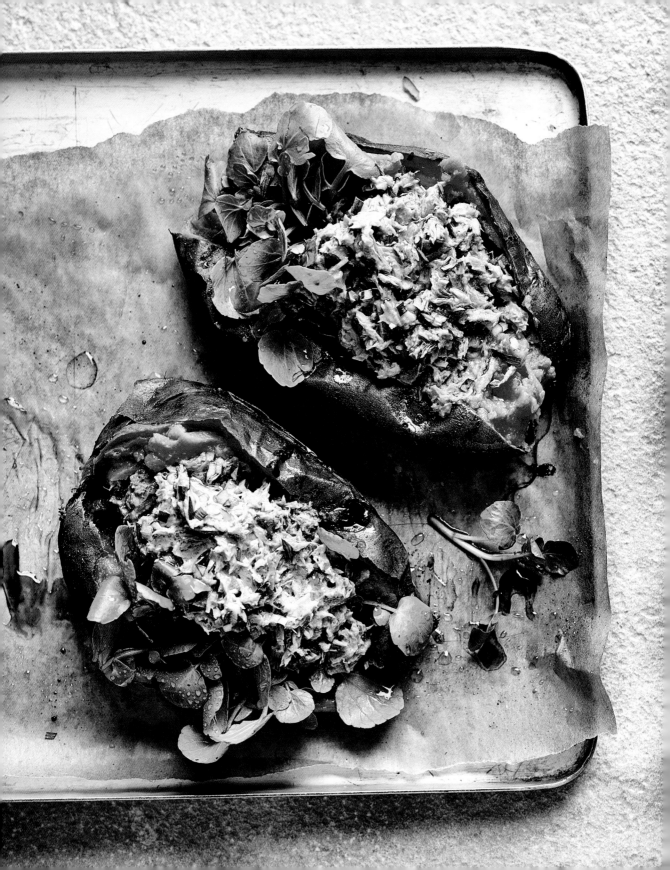

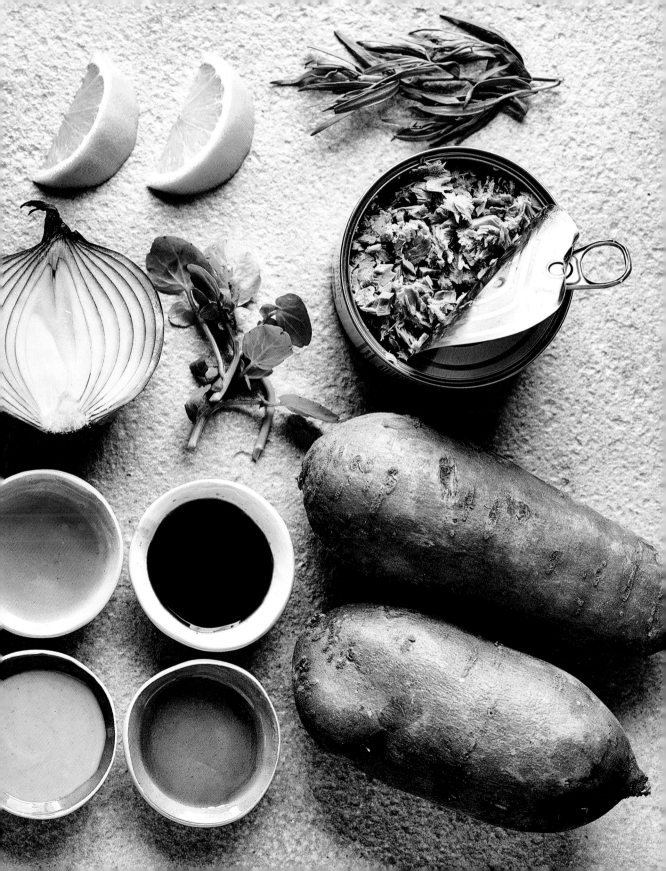

Post-workout dinner plate:
Loaded Sweet Potato Skins, Tuna, Tarragon and Tahini

Try this recipe post-workout for the perfect combination of protein, fats and carbohydrates to refuel and replenish!

2 sweet potatoes (about 300–350g each)
120g tinned tuna, drained
2 tbsp tahini
1 lemon, ½ juiced, ½ sliced into wedges
½ small red onion, peeled, halved and finely chopped
1 tbsp tamari
1 tbsp apple cider vinegar
1 sprig of fresh tarragon, leaves finely chopped, plus extra to serve
2 large handfuls of watercress
extra virgin olive oil, for drizzling
sea salt and freshly ground black pepper

SERVES 2

Cook the sweet potatoes according to the recipe on page 132.

Mix the tuna, tahini, lemon juice, chopped onion, tamari, apple cider vinegar and tarragon in a bowl with 2 tablespoons water until fully combined. Season to taste with salt and pepper.

When the sweet potatoes are cooked, carefully slice into the centre and stuff with the tuna mixture. Sprinkle with the extra tarragon, drizzle with olive oil and serve with the watercress and lemon wedges for squeezing over.

Why this works

After a workout, your body needs a combination of good-quality protein and carbohydrates to help refuel and replenish glycogen levels, and promote recovery. This dinner of tasty tuna and sweet potato provides all of this in one delicious meal, ensuring that you're kept satisfied after your workout!

1. Protein

The predominant source of protein in this meal is tuna, which provides around 28g of protein.

2. Fats

Tahini is a source of essential fatty acids, both omega-3 and omega-6.

3. Carbohydrates

Sweet potato is a nutrient-rich carbohydrate that will keep you satiated.

4. Micronutrients

Watercress is a nutrient-rich green leaf that is an excellent source of vitamin K, while sweet potatoes are an important source of vitamin A and dietary fibre.

More post-workout dinner ideas:

Spicy Baked Butter Beans on Toast (see recipe, page 60), Warm Roasted Butternut Squash, Lentil and Feta Salad with Lemony Tahini Dressing (see recipe, page 94) or Sweet Potato Burgers with Smashed Avocado, Rocket and Parmesan (see recipe, page 204)

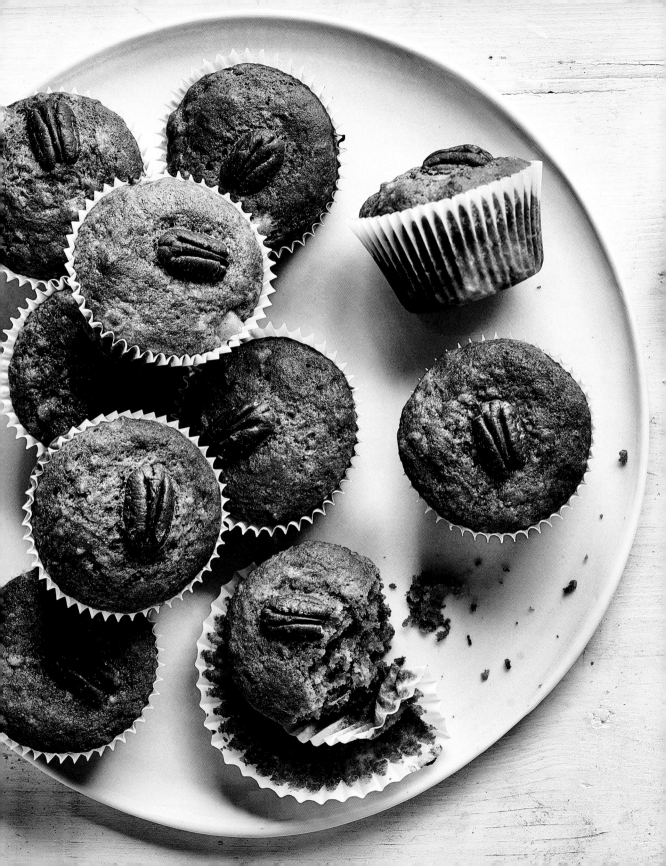

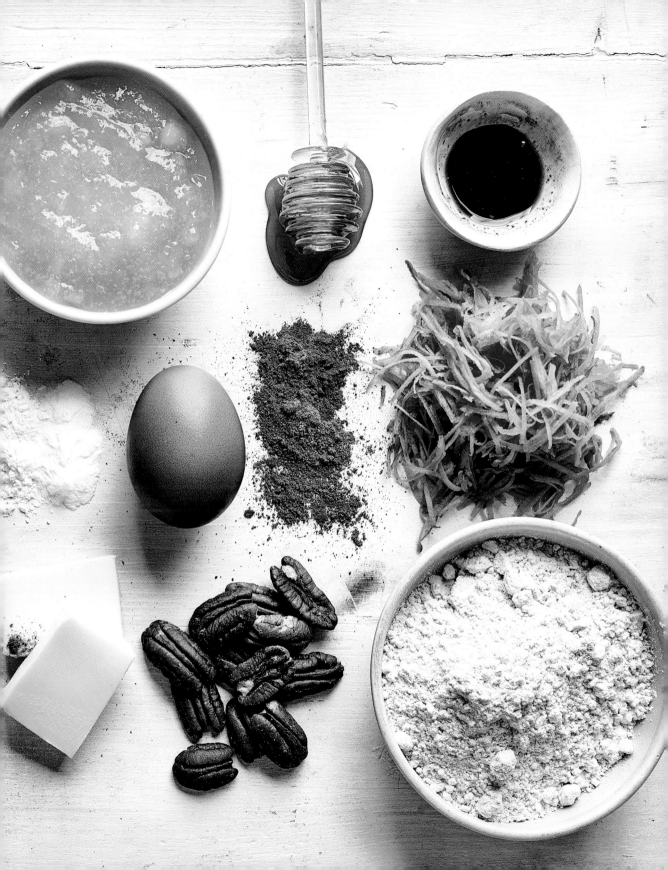

Super snack plate:
Carrot, Apple and Pecan Muffins

(V)

Perfect for weekend baking, and breakfasting in a hurry!

200g spelt flour
1 tsp bicarbonate of soda
1 tsp baking powder
1 tsp ground cinnamon
a generous grating of nutmeg
a pinch of sea salt
30g unsalted butter
150g honey
1 tsp vanilla extract
275g unsweetened apple sauce
1 free-range egg
75g carrot, peeled and grated
12 pecan nuts

MAKES 12

Preheat the oven to 200°C/400°F/Gas Mark 6. Line a muffin tray with 12 paper muffin cases.

In a large mixing bowl, combine the flour, bicarbonate of soda, baking powder, cinnamon, nutmeg and salt.

Place the butter in a small bowl and heat in the microwave until melted.

Make a well in the centre of the flour mixture. Pour in the melted butter, honey, vanilla extract and apple sauce. Crack in the egg and whisk briefly until combined, but don't whisk for too long. Add the grated carrot and whisk again until the mixture is completely combined.

Divide the mixture between the muffin cases and place a pecan on the top of each muffin.

Bake in the hot oven for around 18–20 minutes, or until cooked through, then transfer to a wire rack to cool.

Why this works

Packed full of nutritious goodness, these muffins are the perfect way to satisfy a sweet tooth, and are great for grab-on-the-go snacking for a busy week. With carrots being an excellent source of fibre and vitamin A, these muffins trump the sugar-loaded, shop-bought variety any day.

1. Carbohydrates

These muffins make an excellent alternative to the sugar-loaded, shop-bought versions. Baked with apple sauce and honey, they are a good source of quick energy to the body – which makes them perfect for pre-workout snacking!

2. Micronutrients

Loaded with beta-carotene and vitamin A from the carrots and apple sauce, these muffins are also packed with fibre, which helps to slow the release of sugar into the bloodstream.

More super snack ideas:

Cashew and Kale Crisps (see recipe, page 166), Blueberry Flapjacks (see recipe, page 169) or Spicy Oven-roasted Chickpeas (see recipe, page 168)

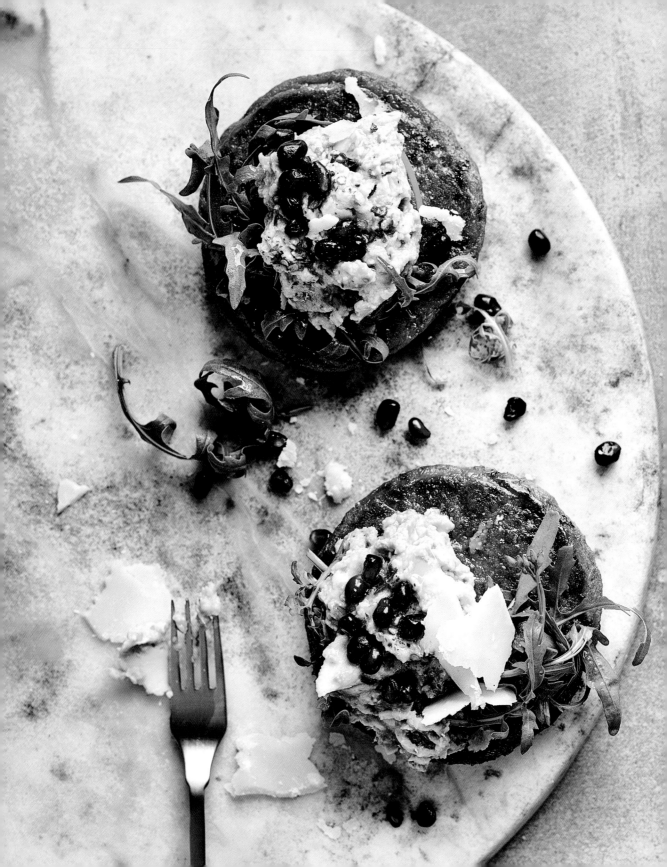

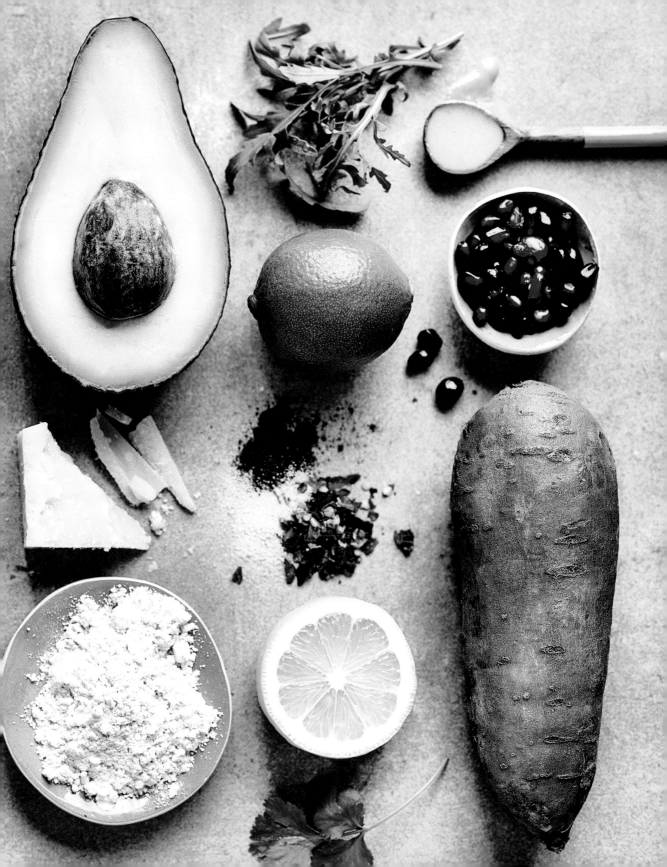

Sunday soul food plate:
Sweet Potato Burgers with Smashed Avocado, Rocket and Parmesan

Okay, we all love burgers, but this veggie twist on the meaty classic is an absolute winner for both meat eaters and veggies alike.

1 large sweet potato, peeled (around 350–400g)

¼ lemon, juiced

1 tsp tahini

¼ tsp chilli flakes

¼ tsp smoked paprika

½ tsp garlic powder

¼ of a bunch of fresh coriander, leaves finely chopped

1 tbsp spelt flour

½ avocado, peeled, halved and stoned

¼ lime, juiced

a pinch of chilli flakes

2 large handfuls of rocket

2 tbsp pomegranate seeds

25g Parmesan cheese

SERVES 2

Preheat the oven to 180°C/350°F/Gas Mark 4. Line a baking tray with greaseproof paper.

Chop the potato into small chunks. Put into a medium saucepan, cover with cold water, bring to the boil, then reduce the heat to low and simmer for 20 minutes, until cooked through. Drain and leave to steam dry.

In a large bowl, mix together the lemon juice, tahini, chilli flakes, smoked paprika, garlic powder, chopped coriander and spelt flour with a pinch of salt and pepper. Add the potato and mash with a potato masher until fully combined.

Once the mixture is cool enough to handle, use your hands to create two burgers. Place on the lined tray and cook in the hot oven for 20 minutes.

Meanwhile, put the avocado flesh into a bowl. Add the lime juice, a little salt and pepper and a pinch of chilli flakes and mash until fully combined.

Serve the burgers with a large handful of rocket. Top with the smashed avocado, sprinkle over the pomegranate seeds and use a vegetable peeler to shave over the Parmesan.

Why this works

There's nothing more satisfying than some serious soul food on a Sunday evening. Now, don't get me wrong, this usually involves some ice cream for me... But for starters, these sweet potato burgers are a pretty perfect end to the weekend. They're also great to cook once and eat twice, so making double of the recipe will ensure you've got a few lunches prepped for the week ahead – a win-win situation!

1. Protein

There is no main source of protein within this dish, but there are some contributory sources – for example, the Parmesan cheese. Avocados also have a higher protein content than many other fruits.

3. Micronutrients

Avocados are also a source of vitamin E which helps protect our bodies against damage.

2. Fats

The avocado in this dish provides an excellent source of healthy fats, with avocados containing heart-healthy monounsaturated fat.

More Sunday soul food ideas:

Dark Chocolate Orange Cookies (see recipe, page 170), Maple Syrup French Toast With Greek Yoghurt and Homemade Strawberry Chia Jam (see recipe, page 54) or Mexican Quinoa Bowl (see recipe, page 152)

MEAL PLANNER

While I never advocate copying or replicating anyone's diet completely, I thought I'd share my weekly meal planner here to show you what a typical week looks like for me. I've done this so that you can see how I structure my meals, giving realistic examples of what I might grab if I'm on the go. The planner also demostrates how I usually cook once and eat twice – so I can prepare some lunches ahead – and what I make if I've got slightly more time. As I've said previously, there isn't a one-size-fits-all approach to nutrition, but I hope my planner helps demonstrate how easy it can be to create a realistic, achievable healthy lifestyle just by incorporating a few small changes.

MONDAY

Breakfast: Mushroom, Spinach and Feta Omelette (see recipe, page 58)

Packed full of protein, this omelette is the perfect way to kick off the week. I always find if I have an omelette to look forward to on a Monday morning, the battle with the bed becomes a little bit easier! I also always look forward to my morning coffee, which I have with a little almond milk nearly every day.

Snack: Beef biltong

I usually have something around 10.30am to tide me over until lunch. I love making my own snacks, but do also pick things up on the go. I often grab some beef biltong from the supermarket, which is one of my all-time favourite treat-time snacks, and an apple. I also love a peppermint tea.

Lunch: Spiced Roast Chicken with Quinoa Tabbouleh (see recipe, page 188)

I usually have my lunch out and about, but will almost always have prepped something in advance to eat. On Mondays I'm often munching on my Sunday dinner leftovers, such as Spiced Roast Chicken with Quinoa Tabbouleh. This dish is so simple to pop into a sealable container and is a great source of both protein and carbohydrates to keep brain function and energy levels high through busy days!

Snack: Greek yoghurt with toppings

By about 3.30pm I usually have a substantial snack, and today's is some Greek yoghurt mixed with fresh berries, toasted oats and seeds. This is such a simple snack to throw together, but really satisfies my sweet tooth and helps me to avoid that afternoon slump!

Dinner: Creamy Puy Lentils with Peas, Feta and Bacon (see recipe, page 126)

Monday's dinner is some serious comfort food. This recipe is the perfect end to the day, with lentils being an awesome source of both starchy carbs and protein and providing a slow release of energy. I make two portions in the evening, and pop half into a sealable container for lunch tomorrow – yum!

Dessert: Brilliant Beetroot Energy Balls (see recipe, page 158)

I always like to have something sweet after dinner and these energy balls are deliciously sweet; they're the perfect way to finish the day!

TUESDAY

Breakfast: Four-Ingredient Banana Pancakes with Warm Berry Compote (see recipe, page 75)

As always, my day starts with my usual coffee. I also have a large glass of cold water before my coffee each morning to rehydrate after sleeping. I find this helps to wake me up! When in a rush I pick a speedy breakfast and this recipe is a quick one. It takes minutes to prep and the pancakes are onto my plate and into my mouth in under 10 minutes. The perfect fuel to kick-start the day!

Snack: Brilliant Beetroot Energy Balls (see recipe, page 158)

When I make a batch of my Brilliant Beetroot Energy Balls, I keep a few in a container in my bag that I snack on at about 11am for a mid morning pick-me-up with a green tea. These store really well if just placed in a sealable container in the fridge, so make for the perfect Sunday meal prep to see you through the week! They're a great bit of pre-workout fuel for my training sessions.

Lunch: Creamy Puy Lentils with Peas, Feta And Bacon (see recipe, page 126)

Last night's leftovers, which I enjoy post workout and wash down with some water, followed by a juicy apple. I am a huge fan of Pink Lady apples, and make sure I get a supply when I do my food shop to see me through the week. Fruit is so dense in nutrients and the perfect sweet treat after a meal, without the added sugar!

Snack: Kale Crisps (see recipe, page 166)

If I'm not feeling too hungry in the afternoon, I'll opt for something like kale crisps. I have an easy recipe for them but there are lots of places that sell them, too. It's great that there are now so many options for delicious healthy snacks when you're out and about!

Dinner: Coriander and Chilli Grilled Chicken Fillets with Smashed Avocado and Wild Rice (see recipe, page 147)

A truly balanced meal, providing good sources of each macronutrient; this is such a tasty way to finish the day!

Dessert: Greek Yoghurt with Toppings

A creature of habit, my dessert is one of my favourite food combinations: some Greek yoghurt with raspberries and a good drizzle of almond butter. My absolute food heaven!

WEDNESDAY

Breakfast: Dippy Eggs with Roasted Parsnip Soldiers (see recipe, page 64)

When I work from home, I spend the majority of my day sitting at a laptop. This doesn't make much of a difference to my food choices, but it does mean I have slightly less of an appetite, as I'm much less active. However, the beauty of working from home means that I have slightly more time to make breakfast, so I'll treat myself to some Dippy Eggs with Parsnip Soldiers – the ultimate combination that is a twist on a childhood favourite!

Snack: Raspberries and toasted almonds

For a light morning snack, a small punnet of fresh raspberries and a small handful of toasted almonds do well. My favourite fruit, raspberries are packed full of goodness, and are the perfect snack to keep me going through the morning. I buy the almonds in big packs and toast them all together in the oven for around 15 minutes or until lightly golden, then store them in a sealable container for a great healthy snack!

Lunch: Quick Butter Bean Tagine with Herby Quinoa (see recipe, page 146)

Lunch today is my quick and simple tagine. Packed full of flavour, I wrote this as a dinner so this is seriously filling, too!

Snack: Date and Almond Energy Balls (see recipe, page 162)

Two of my Date and Almond Energy Balls, which take less than 5 minutes to make. These are seriously scrumptious, but I have to exercise a little portion control or else I could definitely eat about ten!

Dinner: Lemon, Pineapple and Herb-roasted Chicken with Greens (see recipe, page 138)

A protein-packed meal, I save half the recipe for tomorrow – I find this the quickest and simplest way to meal prep without it feeling like a chore!

Dessert: Homemade Blackberry Chia Jam with Greek Yoghurt (see recipe, page 178)

Tonight I'm opting for another simple dessert of Greek yoghurt with some of my homemade blackberry chia jam, which is a delicious sweet treat to finish off the day!

THURSDAY

Breakfast: Chocolate Orange Overnight Oats (see recipe, page 82)

When flying out the door in the morning I grab my 'in a rush' saviour Chocolate Orange Overnight Oats, made the night before, which are the most welcome treat on my morning commute. Although plastic containers aren't glamorous, for those that really struggle for time in the morning this is an excellent option that means you have to quite literally just open the fridge, grab your breakfast and go. Explore different flavour combinations and find your favourite so that you don't find yourself skipping meals.

Snack: Rice cakes and nut butter

Mid morning when I crave something savoury, I pick up some rice cakes and a sachet of nut butter and voilà! – the perfect on-the-go snack! Admittedly, it's not always cheap to buy snacks on the go, but I'm being honest, and showing the quickest and simplest options that I occasionally grab while I'm out.

Lunch: Chicken and quinoa superfood salad (eating out)

Eating out shouldn't be a contentious issue, with so many restaurants and cafés offering delicious healthy dishes. I'm not saying that I don't sometimes opt for something a little more naughty if I fancy it, but usually if it's a general business meeting I try and make good choices like a chicken and quinoa superfood salad, which has loads of veggies, seeds and feta and a lemony dressing, and is absolutely delicious!

Snack: Apple and green tea

My old favourite – a deliciously crunchy Pink Lady washed down with a green tea!

Dinner: Beetroot and Feta Burgers (see recipe, page 153)

My seriously good Beetroot and Feta Burgers taste amazing! I always like spending a little more time on my evening meals, as I have the time to be able to sit and properly enjoy them without rushing off anywhere. These protein-packed, nutrient dense burgers are great for eating alone or entertaining and are such an easy way to make a really impressive meal!

FRIDAY

Breakfast: Chorizo and Feta Mini Egg Muffins (see recipe, page 67)

I usually have a feel-good Friday breakfast to end the week on a high. My Chorizo and Feta Mini Egg Muffins are so simple and quick to prepare and are packed full of flavour. Serve with some grilled asparagus and chopped fresh spinach for some added greens.

Snack: Chocolate Chia Smoothie (see recipe, page 176)

For a post-workout snack, I opt for my Chocolate Chia Smoothie and add a scoop of chocolate whey to aid muscle recovery. I try to make my recipes as versatile as possible, and simply adding a scoop of whey to this smoothie provides a great post-workout refuel!

Lunch: Beetroot and Feta Burgers (see recipe, page 153)

As repetitive as I feel I sound, I'll munch into the dinner I made the night before for lunch (which is why a lot of my recipes serve 2). Although it may feel weird, it soon becomes habit and saves time and money when you might have bought food on the go or eaten out!

Snack: Veggies and Courgette Hummus

Chopped veggies such as carrots, celery and cucumber with some homemade Courgette Hummus (recipe in *The Body Bible*). This is a deliciously simple snack that takes minimum effort and stores well in the fridge for a few days, for the perfect go-to snack when you're feeling peckish!

Dinner: Venison Steak with Soy, Pomegranate and Ginger and Miso-glazed Parsnip Fries (see recipe, page 120)

I'm finishing the week with a bit of a treat of Venison Steak with Soy, Pomegranate and Ginger and some Miso-glazed Parsnip Fries.

Dessert: Date and Almond Energy Balls (see recipe, page 162)

It's Friday night, and I'm often feeling indulgent, so I'll create a bowl full of yumminess with two of my Energy Balls, some ice cream and crumbled dark chocolate! I can't express how important it is to incorporate this kind of balance into your week. As you can see, I would've eaten well for the whole week and felt great, but I'm not going to restrict myself from having the occasional sugary treat either. In my opinion, it's essential not to see any food as bad, or banned, which is beneficial to both body and mind.

SATURDAY

Breakfast: Smoked Salmon and Dill Omelette with Spiced Greek Yoghurt (see recipe, page 59)

With a slightly slower pace to my weekends, breakfasts are the meal I look forward to most. This is such a classic combo, with a nice flavoursome twist, and although I certainly couldn't afford to be eating smoked salmon every day, a cheeky weekend foodie splurge is totally worth every penny!

Snack: Spicy Oven-roasted Chickpeas (see recipe, page 168)

A pre-workout snack for a bit of an energy boost. These are a really cheap and easy snack to make, have a great nutritional profile and also taste really good! Try roasting a big batch on a Sunday evening when you have a little more time and store them for easy snacks throughout the week.

Lunch: Scrambled eggs on rye toast

For a post-workout lunch, I have some good and simple scrambled eggs on rye toast. This provides a perfect balance of protein and carbohydrate to refuel me after my gym session!

Snack: Apple, nut butter and toasted almonds

A snack of choice for an afternoon of socialising with friends is some fresh apple (can you tell I love apples?) sliced with some nut butter drizzled over and a few toasted almonds.

Dinner: Cashew, Carrot, Pomegranate and Halloumi Salad (see recipe, page 150)

I am a huge fan of cheese, and halloumi is up there as one of my favourites. This salad has the most delicious dressing, too!

Dessert: Homemade Blackberry Chia Jam with Greek Yoghurt (see recipe, page 178)

Dessert is often super simple Greek yoghurt with my homemade blackberry chia jam!

SUNDAY

Breakfast: Maple Syrup French Toast with Greek Yoghurt and Homemade Strawberry Chia Jam (see recipe, page 54)

The absolute sweet treat of my French toast is seriously one of my all-time favourite breakfasts and is perfect for a lazy Sunday morning!

Lunch: Salmon, Seeds, Avocado and Dill (see recipe, page 90)

After quite a big and filling breakfast I'd skip a morning snack, opting for some simple salmon with avocado, seeds and dill for lunch. I always try to eat at least one portion of oily fish throughout the week to ensure that I'm getting enough omega-3s into my diet.

Snack: Frozen raspberries

Don't knock it until you've tried it. I love apples, but frozen berries are perfect to store without getting damaged and are ideal for easy snacking.

Dinner: Everyday Chicken with Roasted Butternut Squash, Lime and Chilli (see recipe, page 134)

I absolutely love entertaining and cooking for others. My Everyday Chicken is the perfect dish for cooking on a larger scale and is always a hit with my family!

Dessert: Date and Almond Energy Balls (see recipe, page 162)

To finish my evening, I tuck into a couple of energy balls with a handful of fresh raspberries and a little bit of dark chocolate! The perfect way to finish the week!

Conversion Charts

DRY WEIGHTS

METRIC	IMPERIAL	METRIC	IMPERIAL
5g	¼oz	500g	1lb 2oz
8/10g	⅓oz	550g	1lb 3oz
15g	½oz	600g	1lb 5oz
20g	¾oz	625g	1lb 6oz
25g	1oz	650g	1lb 7oz
30/35g	1¼oz	675g	1½lb
40g	1½oz	700g	1lb 9oz
50g	2oz	750g	1lb 10oz
60/70g	2½oz	800g	1¾lb
75/85/90g	3oz	850g	1lb 14oz
100g	3½oz	900g	2lb
110/120g	4oz	950g	2lb 2oz
125/130g	4½oz	1kg	2lb 3oz
135/140/150g	5oz	1.1kg	2lb 6oz
170/175g	6oz	1.25kg	2¾lb
200g	7oz	1.3/1.4kg	3lb
225g	8oz	1.5kg	3lb 5oz
250g	9oz	1.75/1.8kg	4lb
265g	9½oz	2kg	4lb 4oz
275g	10oz	2.25kg	5lb
300g	11oz	2.5kg	5½lb
325g	11½oz	3kg	6½lb
350g	12oz	3.5kg	7¾lb
375g	13oz	4kg	8¾lb
400g	14oz	4.5kg	9¾lb
425g	15oz	6.8kg	15lb
450g	1lb	9kg	20lb
475g	1lb 1oz		

568ml = 1 UK pint (20fl oz) | 16fl oz = 1 US pint

LIQUID MEASURES

METRIC	IMPERIAL	CUPS	METRIC	IMPERIAL	CUPS
15ml	½fl oz	1 tbsp (level)	425ml	15fl oz	
20ml	¾fl oz		450ml	16fl oz	2 cups
25ml	1fl oz	⅛ cup	500ml	18fl oz	2¼ cups
30ml	1¼fl oz		550ml	19fl oz	
50ml	2fl oz	¼ cup	600ml	1 pint	2½ cups
60ml	2½fl oz		700ml	1¼ pints	
75ml	3fl oz		750ml	1⅓ pints	
100ml	3½fl oz	⅜ cup	800ml	1 pint 9fl oz	
110/120ml	4fl oz	½ cup	850ml	1½ pints	
125ml	4½fl oz		900ml	1 pint 12fl oz	3¾ cups
150ml	5fl oz	⅔ cup	1 litre	1¾ pints	1 US quart (4 cups)
175ml	6fl oz	¾ cup	1.2 litres	2 pints	1¼ US quarts
200/215ml	7fl oz		1.25 litres	2¼ pints	
225ml	8fl oz	1 cup	1.5 litres	2½ pints	3 US pints
250ml	9fl oz		1.75/1.8 litres	3 pints	
275ml	9½fl oz		2 litres	3½ pints	2 US quarts
300ml	½ pint	1¼ cups	2.2 litres	3¾ pints	
350ml	12fl oz	1½ cups	2.5 litres	4⅓ pints	
375ml	13fl oz		3 litres	5 pints	
400ml	14fl oz		3.5 litres	6 pints	

OVEN TEMPERATURES

All recipes are based on fan-assisted oven temperatures. If you are using a conventional oven,
raise the temperature 20°C higher than stated in recipes.

°C	°F	GAS MARK	DESCRIPTION
110	225	¼	cool
130	250	½	cool
140	275	1	very low
150	300	2	very low
160/170	325	3	low to moderate
180	350	4	moderate
190	375	5	moderately hot
200	400	6	hot
220	425	7	hot
230	450	8	hot
240	475	9	very hot

Index

Page references in *italics* denote photographs.

A

Asian-style Shredded Rainbow Veggie Noodle Salad *144*, 145

aubergines
Mini Turkey Burger and Aubergine Bites 99
Roasted Aubergine with Feta, Tahini, Pomegranate and Yoghurt 106, *107*

avocados
Blueberry and Avocado Breakfast Muffins 86, *87*
Kale, Avocado and Citrus Smoothie 174, *175*
Salmon, Seeds, Avocado and Dill 90, *91*, 193, 215

B

bananas
Chocolate and Banana Protein Power Oats 83
Four-ingredient Banana Pancakes with Warm Berry Compote *74*, 75, 210
Super Simple Banana and Blueberry Loaf 163

beetroot
Beetroot and Feta Burgers 153, 212, 213
Beetroot and Feta Frittata *68*, 69
Brilliant Beetroot Energy Balls 158, *160–1*, 209, 210
Super Simple Beetroot Crisps 167

blueberries
Blueberry and Avocado Breakfast Muffins 86, *87*
Blueberry Flapjacks 169, 201
Super Simple Banana and Blueberry Loaf 163

breakfast 52–87

Breakfast Wrap with Homemade Chunky Salsa, Ultimate 72, *73*

broccoli
Citrus Baked Salmon with Broccoli Pesto 137
Maple Syrup and Pistachio-crusted Salmon with Tenderstem Broccoli 124
Poached Eggs with Broccoli, Feta, Chilli and Garlic 62
Souper Simple Broccoli Soup 98, 193
Sweet Potato and Tenderstem Broccoli Frittata 114

burgers
Beetroot and Feta Burgers 153, 212, 213
Mini Turkey Burger and Aubergine Bites 99
Spicy Salmon Burgers with Courgetti *190–1*, 192, 193
Sweet Potato Burgers with Smashed Avocado, Rocket and Parmesan 197, *202–3*, 204, 205
Thai-style Turkey Burgers *96*, 97, 189

butter beans
Quick Butter Bean Tagine with Herby Quinoa 146, 211
Spicy Baked Butter Beans on Toast 60, *61*, 197

butternut squash
Butternut Squash and Quinoa Chilli 100, *101*
Everyday Chicken with Roasted Butternut Squash, Lime and Chilli 134, *135*, 215
Warm Roasted Butternut Squash, Lentil and Feta Salad with Lemony Tahini Dressing 94, 197

C

Caramel Slices, Raw Salted 156, *157*

carbohydrates 42

carrots
Carrot, Apple and Pecan Muffins *198–9*, 200, 201
Cashew, Carrot, Pomegranate and Halloumi Salad 150, *151*, 214

cashews
Cashew and Kale Crisps 166, 201
Cashew, Carrot, Pomegranate and Halloumi Salad 150, *151*, 214
Chewy Coconut, Cashew and Chia Bars 179

Ceviche, Salmon and Mango 112, *113*

chia
Chewy Coconut, Cashew and Chia Bars 179
Chocolate Chia Smoothie 176, *177*, 213
Coconut and Fig Overnight Chia Pudding 76, *77*
Homemade Blackberry Chia Jam with Greek Yoghurt 178, 211, 214
Maple Syrup French Toast with Greek Yoghurt and Homemade Strawberry Chia Jam 54, *55*, 205, 215

chicken
Chilli and Lime Chicken with Grilled Tomatoes and Guacamole 125
Coriander and Chilli Grilled Chicken Fillets with Smashed Avocado and Wild Rice 147, 210
Everyday Chicken with Roasted Butternut Squash, Lime and Chilli 134, *135*, 215
Lemon, Pineapple and Herb-roasted Chicken with Greens 138, *139*, 211

Spiced Roast Chicken with
Quinoa Tabbouleh *186–7*,
188, 189, 209
Wild Rice, Roasted Chickpea
and Harissa Chicken Salad
116, *117*
chickpeas
Spicy Oven-roasted Chickpeas
168, 201, 214
Vanilla Chickpea Energy Balls
159, *160–1*
Wild Rice, Roasted Chickpea
and Harissa Chicken Salad
116, *117*
Chilli, Butternut Squash and Quinoa
100, *101*
chillies
Chilli and Lime Chicken
with Grilled Tomatoes and
Guacamole 125
Coriander and Chilli Grilled
Chicken Fillets with Smashed
Avocado and Wild Rice 147,
210
chocolate
Chocolate and Banana Protein
Power Oats 83
Chocolate Chia Smoothie 176,
177, 213
Chocolate Orange Overnight
Oats 82, 212
Dark Chocolate Orange Cookies
170, *171*, 205
Chorizo and Feta Mini Egg Muffins
67, 213
citrus
Citrus Baked Salmon with
Broccoli Pesto 137
Citrus Roasted Root Veg with
Gooey Goat's Cheese 142, *143*
Kale, Avocado and Citrus
Smoothie 174, *175*
coconuts
Chewy Coconut, Cashew and
Chia Bars 179

Coconut and Almond Butter
Cookies *171*, 172
Coconut and Fig Overnight Chia
Pudding 76, *77*
Creamy Coconut Oats with Kiwi
and Almond Butter 79
Oatmeal Cookie Sandwiches
with Coconut and Lemon
Cashew Cream *171*, 173
Raspberry and Coconut
Breakfast Loaf 84, *85*
cod
Homemade Pesto Courgetti with
Baked Cod 109
Kale Pesto-baked Cod 128
Spiced Cod with Turmeric
Roasted Cauliflower 148, *149*
conversion charts 216, 217
cookies
Coconut and Almond Butter
Cookies *171*, 172
Dark Chocolate Orange Cookies
170, *171*, 205
Oatmeal Cookie Sandwiches
with Coconut and Lemon
Cashew Cream *171*, 173
Coriander and Chilli Grilled Chicken
Fillets with Smashed Avocado and
Wild Rice 147, 210
courgettes
Crispy Courgette Fritters with
Smoked Salmon 56, *57*
Homemade Pesto Courgetti with
Baked Cod 109
Spicy Salmon Burgers with
Courgetti *190–1*, 192, 193
crisps
Cashew and Kale Crisps 166, 201
Super Simple Beetroot Crisps 167

D
Date and Almond Energy Balls *160–1*,
162, 211, 213, 215
dinner 118–53

E
eggs
Chorizo and Feta Mini Egg
Muffins 67, 213
Dippy Eggs with Roasted
Parsnip Soldiers 64, *65*, 211
Fried Eggs with Quinoa, Kale,
Pomegranate and Pumpkin
Seeds 63
Poached Eggs with Broccoli,
Feta, Chilli and Garlic 62
energy balls
Brilliant Beetroot Energy Balls
158, *160–1*, 209, 210
Date and Almond Energy Balls
160–1, 162, 211, 213, 215
Vanilla Chickpea Energy Balls
159, *160–1*
exercise 16

F
fats 43
feta
Beetroot and Feta Burgers 153,
212, 213
Beetroot and Feta Frittata *68*, 69
Chorizo and Feta Mini Egg
Muffins 67, 213
Mushroom, Spinach and Feta
Omelette 58, 185, 209
Warm Roasted Butternut
Squash, Lentil and Feta Salad
with Lemony Tahini Dressing
94, 197
fibre, dietary 46–7
first week 14–17
Flapjacks, Blueberry 169, 201
frittata
Beetroot and Feta Frittata *68*, 69
Full English Breakfast Frittata 66
Sweet Potato and Tenderstem
Broccoli Frittata 114

G
goals, setting 26, 27

goat's cheese
    Citrus Roasted Root Veg with
        Gooey Goat's Cheese 142, *143*
    Gooey Goat's Cheese Scramble
        in Portobello Mushrooms 108
    Gooey Goat's Cheese, Tomato
        and Rocket Omelette *182–3*,
        184, 185
    Loaded Sweet Potato Skins
        (Roasted Fig, Honey and
        Goat's Cheese) 133
    Super Seed Loaf with Goat's
        Cheese and Grilled Tomatoes
        104
Greek yoghurt 209, 210
    Greek Yoghurt with Warm
        Cinnamon-spiced Stewed
        Blueberry and Apple 78
    Homemade Blackberry Chia Jam
        with Greek Yoghurt 178, 211, 214
    Maple Syrup French Toast with
        Greek Yoghurt and
        Homemade Strawberry Chia
        Jam 54, *55*, 205, 215
    Smoked Salmon and Dill
        Omelette with Spiced Greek
        Yoghurt 59, 214

H
harissa
    Harissa and Lime Salmon
        Parcels with Coconut Rice
        130, 131
    Wild Rice, Roasted Chickpea
        and Harissa Chicken Salad
        116, *117*

K
kale
    Cashew and Kale Crisps 166, 201
    Fried Eggs with Quinoa, Kale,
        Pomegranate and Pumpkin
        Seeds 63
    Kale, Avocado and Citrus
        Smoothie 174, *175*
    Kale Pesto-baked Cod 128

L
lentils
    Creamy Puy Lentils with Peas,
        Feta and Bacon 126, *127*, 209,
        210
    Griddled Steak with Balsamic
        Puy Lentils and Feta 136
    Warm Roasted Butternut
        Squash, Lentil and Feta Salad
        with Lemony Tahini Dressing
        94, 197
lunch 88–117

M
mackerel
    Loaded Sweet Potato Skins
        (Smoked Mackerel, Yoghurt
        and Dill) 132
    Smoked Mackerel with Wilted
        Spinach and Avocado 70
    Spicy Smoked Mackerel on
        Toast 71
macronutrients 38–9
mangoes
    Mango and Lime 'Slushie' 174, *175*
    Salmon and Mango Ceviche 112, *113*
maple syrup
    Maple Syrup and Pistachio-
        crusted Salmon with
        Tenderstem Broccoli 124
    Maple Syrup French Toast with
        Greek Yoghurt and Homemade
        Strawberry Chia Jam 54, *55*,
        205, 215
meal planner 206–15
Mexican Quinoa Bowl 152, 205
micronutrients 44–5
mind 17
morning routine 24, 25
muffins
    Blueberry and Avocado
        Breakfast Muffins 86, *87*
    Carrot, Apple and Pecan Muffins
        198–9, 200, 201
    Chorizo and Feta Mini Egg
        Muffins 67, 213

mushrooms
    Gooey Goat's Cheese
        Scramble in Portobello
        Mushrooms 108
    Mushroom and Mozzarella
        Shakshuka 110, *111*
    Mushroom, Spinach and Feta
        Omelette 58, 185, 209

N
nutrition 36–49

O
Oatmeal Cookie Sandwiches with
    Coconut and Lemon Cashew
    Cream *171*, 173
oats
    Chocolate and Banana Protein
        Power Oats 83
    Chocolate Orange Overnight
        Oats 82, 212
    Creamy Coconut Oats with Kiwi
        and Almond Butter 79
    Vanilla Overnight Oats with a
        Sweet Strawberry Sauce 82
    Vanilla, Plum and Pistachio
        Power Oats 80, *81*
omelettes
    Gooey Goat's Cheese, Tomato
        and Rocket Omelette *182–3*,
        184, 185
    Mushroom, Spinach and Feta
        Omelette 58, 185, 209
    Smoked Salmon and Dill
        Omelette with Spiced Greek
        Yoghurt 59, 214

P
Pancakes, Four-ingredient Banana with
    Warm Berry Compote *74*, 75, 210
plates 180–205
Prawn Skewers, Griddled with a
    Harissa and Honey Dressing
    122, *123*
Promise, The 34–5
protein 41

Q

quinoa

Butternut Squash and Quinoa Chilli 100, *101*

Fried Eggs with Quinoa, Kale, Pomegranate and Pumpkin Seeds 63

Mexican Quinoa Bowl 152, 205

Quick Butter Bean Tagine with Herby Quinoa 146, 211

Spiced Roast Chicken with Quinoa Tabbouleh *186–7*, 188, 189, 209

R

Raspberry and Coconut Breakfast Loaf 84, *85*

realistic, be 32–3

recipes 50–205

rice

Coriander and Chilli Grilled Chicken Fillets with Smashed Avocado and Wild Rice 147, 210

Harissa and Lime Salmon Parcels with Coconut Rice *130*, 131

Wild Rice, Roasted Chickpea and Harissa Chicken Salad 116, *117*

S

salads

Asian-style Shredded Rainbow Veggie Noodle *144*, 145

Cashew, Carrot, Pomegranate and Halloumi Salad 150, *151*, 214

Green and Lean Super Salad with Creamy Cashew Dressing 129

Shredded Sprout, Bacon and Almond Salad 95, 193

Warm Roasted Butternut Squash, Lentil and Feta Salad with Lemony Tahini Dressing 94, 197

Wild Rice, Roasted Chickpea and Harissa Chicken Salad 116, *117*

salmon

Citrus Baked Salmon with Broccoli Pesto 137

Crispy Courgette Fritters with Smoked Salmon 56, *57*

Harissa and Lime Salmon Parcels with Coconut Rice *130*, 131

Maple Syrup and Pistachio-crusted Salmon with Tenderstem Broccoli 124

Salmon and Mango Ceviche 112, *113*

Salmon, Seeds, Avocado and Dill 90, *91*, 193, 215

Smoked Salmon and Dill Omelette with Spiced Greek Yoghurt 59, 214

Spicy Salmon Burgers with Courgetti *190–1*, 192, 193

Super Seed Loaf with Smoked Salmon and Minted Yoghurt 105

Shakshuka, Mushroom and Mozzarella 110, *111*

'Slushie', Mango and Lime 174, *175*

smoothies

Chocolate Chia Smoothie 176, *177*, 213

Kale, Avocado and Citrus Smoothie 174, *175*

Super Strawberry Crush 164, *165*

snacks 154–79

Soup, Souper Simple Broccoli 98, 193

Sprout, Bacon and Almond Salad, Shredded 95, 193

steak

Griddled Steak with Balsamic Puy Lentils and Feta 136

Steak and Balsamic Caramelised Red Onion Wrap 92, *93*

Venison Steak with Soy, Pomegranate and Ginger and Miso-glazed Parsnip Fries 120, *121*, 213

Strawberry Crush Smoothie, Super 164, *165*

sugar 48–9

Super Seed Loaf 102, *102, 103*

Super Seed Loaf with Goat's

Cheese and Grilled Tomatoes 104

Super Seed Loaf with Smoked Salmon and Minted Yoghurt 105

swaps, make simple 28–31

sweet potatoes

Loaded Sweet Potato Skins, Tuna, Tarragon and Tahini *194–5*, 196, 197

Loaded Sweet Potato Skins Two Ways 132, 133

Sweet Potato and Tenderstem Broccoli Frittata 114

Sweet Potato Burgers with Smashed Avocado, Rocket and Parmesan 197, *202–3*, 204, 205

T

turkey

Mini Turkey Burger and Aubergine Bites 99

Thai Turkey Stir-fry with Chilli and Basil 140, *141*

Thai-style Turkey Burgers *96*, 97, 189

V

vanilla

Vanilla Chickpea Energy Balls 159, *160–1*

Vanilla Overnight Oats with a Sweet Strawberry Sauce 82

Vanilla, Plum and Pistachio Power Oats 80, *81*

Veg with Gooey Goat's Cheese, Citrus Roasted Root 142, *143*

Veggie Noodle Salad, Asian-style Shredded Rainbow *144*, 145

Veggie Slaw, Shredded with Avocado and Sunflower Seeds 115

Venison Steak with Soy, Pomegranate and Ginger and Miso-glazed Parsnip Fries 120, *121*, 213

Acknowledgements

First, I would like to say a huge thank you to my mum – my number one cheerleader, biggest fan and avid follower who has helped me every step of the way to produce this book. Without her help, guidance and constant shoulder to cry on in times of stress, I wouldn't be where I am today.

I'd also like to thank my amazing team at HarperCollins; my publisher, Carolyn Thorne, and everyone who has helped to bring this book to life and put my dreams into reality on the page – I couldn't be more grateful for your continued support! Also to Martin, Kim and the incredible team who shot every photo for this book – we had a vision and we nailed it. I thank you for every painstaking adjustment of each rocket leaf to finally capture what I feel are some pretty amazing shots.

Thanks, too, to my friends and the rest of my family for continuing to keep me smiling every day and for always being there to try my recipe successes (and failures) – and give me feedback along the way!

To Carly Cook, for believing in my vision from day one and helping me through the highs and lows that I've gone through while writing this book. Without Carly, I simply wouldn't have achieved even half of what I have done and I am eternally grateful for her support, honesty and, above all, friendship.

Finally – and most importantly – thanks to you guys, the reason why I have had the incredible opportunity to create this book. From the very beginning it has been you who have inspired, motivated and driven me to achieve all I have done, and I want to thank every single one of you who takes the time to read and use this book. I hope you love using it as much as I loved creating it.

Big love, and even bigger thanks,

Alice x

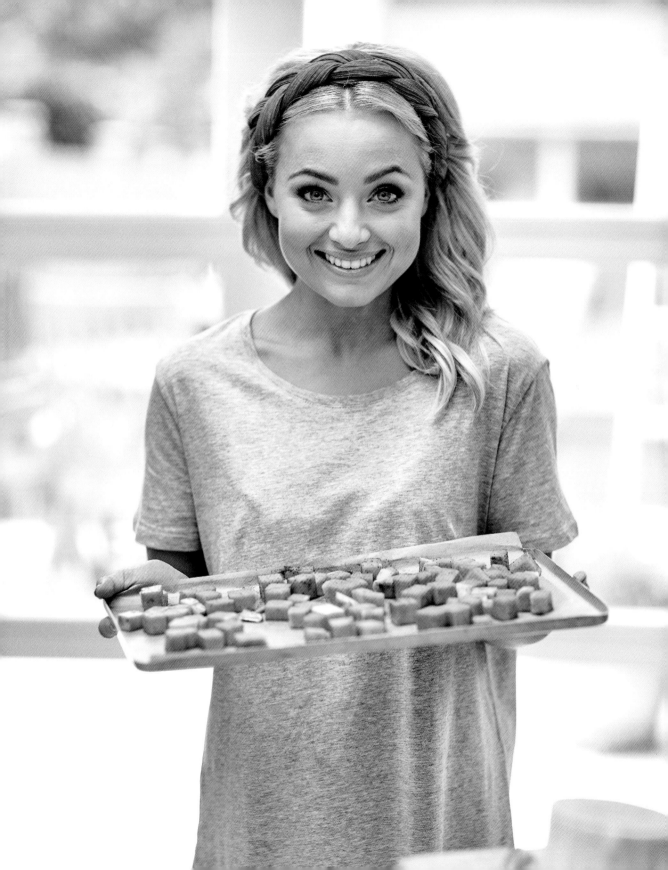

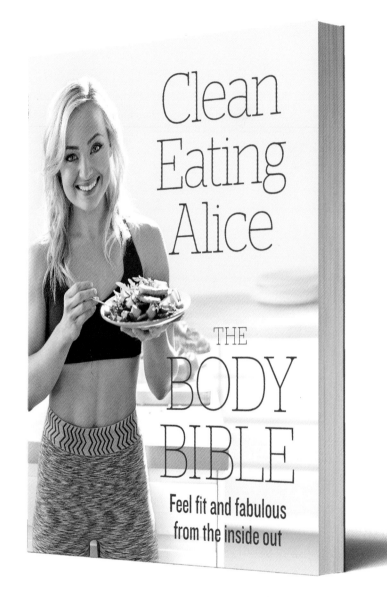

ALSO AVAILABLE